Assisted Human Reproduction

Assisted Human Reproduction

Psychological and Ethical Dilemmas

Edited by

DANI SINGER DipPsych, MA Psych and Couns, UKCP/BACP
Psychotherapist and Counsellor, Northwick Park Hospital
London

and

MYRA HUNTER PhD
Consultant Clinical Psychologist, South London and Maudsley NHS Trust,
and Honorary Senior Lecturer, Guy's, King's and St Thomas'
Schools of Medicine, London

W
WHURR PUBLISHERS
LONDON AND PHILADELPHIA

© 2003 Whurr Publishers Ltd
First published 2003
by Whurr Publishers Ltd
19b Compton Terrace
London N1 2UN England and
325 Chestnut Street, Philadelphia PA 19106 USA

Reprinted 2004

British Library Cataloguing in Publication Data

A catalogue record for this book
is available from the British Library.

ISBN 1 86156 349 3

Printed and bound in the UK by Athenaeum Press Ltd, Gateshead,
Tyne & Wear.

Contents

Contributors

Eric Blyth MA, PhD, CQSW, Professor of Social Work, University of Huddersfield, UK

Ken Daniels, Associate Professor, Department of Social Work, University of Canterbury, New Zealand

Julia Feast MA, CQSW, The Children's Society Post Adoption and Care Counselling Research Project, London, UK

Myra Hunter PhD, Consultant Clinical Psychologist, South London and Maudsley NHS Trust, and Honorary Senior Lecturer, Guy's, King's and St Thomas' Schools of Medicine, London, UK

Robert G Lee, Professor of Law, Cardiff Law School, and Co-Director, ESRC Centre for Business, Relationships, Accountability, Sustainability and Society

Alexina M McWhinnie Cert in Social Studies, MA, PhD, Cert Psychiatric Social Work, Counsellor and Senior Research Fellow, University of Dundee, UK

Nina Martin BSc, PhD, Research Student, University of Huddersfield, UK

Derek Morgan, Professor of Health Care Law, Cardiff Law School, UK and Visiting Senior Fellow, Melbourne Law School, Australia

Clare Murray, PhD, Senior Research Psychologist, Family and Child Psychology Research Centre, City University, London, UK

Sharon A Pettle MSc, DClinPsychol, Consultant Clinical Psychologist and UKCP Systemic Psychotherapist, Donor Conception Project, Centre for Applied Social and Psychological Development, Salomons, part of the Canterbury Christ Church University College, Kent and the Hospital for Sick Children, London, UK

Claire Potter BSc, PhD, Research Student, University of Huddersfield, UK

Jim Richards MA Public and Social Administration, Senior Social Worker, Director, Catholic Children's Society, Westminster, London, UK

Françoise Shenfield LRCP, MRCS, MA, Clinical Lecturer in Obstetrics and Gynaecology, Reproductive Medicine Unit, University College Hospital, London, and Honorary Lecturer in Medicine (Medical Law and Ethics), University College London Medical School, London, UK

Dani Singer DipPsych, MA Psych and Couns, UKCP/BACP, Psychotherapist and Counsellor, Northwick Park Hospital, London, UK

Foreword

This book brings together key commentators on social and ethical issues in the field of assisted reproduction to produce a timely and informative account of some of the most pressing issues facing us today. A particularly appealing and worthwhile feature is that the authors come from a range of backgrounds and thus provide the reader with an all-round perspective of the various topics discussed. Whether new to the field or a veteran, this book will give the reader new insights into the complex issues that arise from the practice of different assisted reproduction procedures and the consequences for all the parties concerned. By taking a broad and long-term view, the multifaceted implications for individuals, families and society as a whole are presented in a fresh light to increase understanding of issues that are of fundamental importance to us all.

In Chapter 1, Eric Blyth and colleagues integrate a historical account of the formation of the Human Fertilisation and Embryology Act 1990, with a discussion of key social and ethical issues that arise from its implementation. They highlight the vagueness of the requirement that account should be taken of the welfare of any child who may be born as a result of treatment, and point to a tendency for greater weight to be placed on the marital status and sexual orientation of prospective parents than on other aspects of parenting. They also focus on the differential access to treatment services that exists according to geographical location and the ability to pay, and the limitations associated with the provision of infertility counselling, including the contradictions involved in combining independent counselling with the screening of potential parents. In their discussion of surrogacy and posthumous conception, they alert the reader to inadequacies in current legislation. They also tackle the controversial topics of payment to gamete donors, access to information about gamete donors, and the nature of the relationship between the Human Fertilisation Embryology Authority (HFEA) and licensed clinics.

Françoise Shenfield focuses on two key issues in Chapter 2: gamete donation and sex selection. With respect to gamete donation, she presents the differing opinions and arguments for and against the payment of gamete donors. She also tackles the controversial issue of egg sharing and highlights the ethical problems that arise. Finally, she considers what kind of non-identifying information about donors should be available to donor offspring and whether or not donor identification may be desirable from the perspective of the different parties involved. Shenfield discusses these issues in the context of legislation on human rights. With regard to sex selection, she presents the opposing views on sex selection for social reasons and argues that, whatever the reason for sex selection, such a practice devalues the position of women.

Jim Richards, in Chapter 3, gives an account of different religious perspectives on a range of issues raised by the practice of assisted human reproduction and embryo research. He highlights similarities and differences among the major faiths with particular attention to artificial insemination by husband, third-party reproduction, *in vitro* fertilization and surrogacy. These issues are discussed in the context of the views of the major religions about the role of marriage, the status of the human embryo and the fundamental question of when human life begins. He lays out the arguments against practices such as surrogacy, human cloning and techniques that involve the destruction of spare embryos, and outlines some of the major religions' criticisms of the Warnock Report and the HFEA.

Theoretical debates that arise from the practice of assisted reproduction from a human rights' perspective are considered by Derek Morgan and Robert Lee in Chapter 4, with particular attention to the right to procreative autonomy. The authors describe three cases in the UK that fall under the Human Rights Act 1998. The first concerns a prisoner who wished his wife to be artificially inseminated with his sperm, the second represents a challenge to the law on the identification of gamete donors, and the third relates to use of genetic testing to enable a child to be born whose cells may be used to save the life of an older brother. The authors discuss these cases in the context of the Human Rights Act, highlighting differing interpretations that may be made. They conclude that developments in assisted reproduction will continue to present challenges in relation to human rights.

In Chapter 5, Julia Feast examines the similarities and differences between donor-assisted conception and adoption with respect to the law, and the implications for those born as a result of donor conception. Drawing from her own research she describes the feelings and experiences of adopted children and adults, and the importance of information about birth parents for the development of a secure sense of identity. Although acknowledging the difficulties presented by openness, she emphasizes that telling children does not have an adverse effect on their relationship with their adoptive parents, and that it is the adoptive parents who are viewed as the real parents. Based on the experiences of adopted children and adults, Feast argues for openness by donor insemination parents and a change in legislation to allow donor identification. She also points to a need for ways of helping parents to be open with children about their donor conception.

Clare Murray, in Chapter 6, examines empirical evidence on the quality of parenting and the psychological well-being of children in assisted reproduction families in relation to the concerns that have been expressed. She concludes that traditional, two-parent, assisted reproduction families, whether created by *in vitro* fertilization, egg donation or donor insemination, appear to be functioning well, with no evidence of raised levels of psychological difficulties among the children. The same appears to be true of children raised in two-parent lesbian mother families. She stresses, however, that little is known about the outcomes for mothers and children when single women have children through donor insemination. Murray also highlights the finding that many heterosexual parents of children conceived by gamete donation do not tell children about their donor conception. In contrast, lesbian mothers are much more likely to be open with their children about this issue. She points out that the situation regarding the secrecy or openness of single heterosexual mothers is as yet unknown.

Alexina McWhinnie explores a number of ethical issues raised by the practice of assisted human reproduction in Chapter 7, including the dilemmas faced by parents whose religious beliefs are incompatible with the method by which they had a child, the problems that result from multiple births with respect to the physical, psychological and financial costs for the families involved, and the negative consequences of foetal reduction where parents opt to reduce a multiple pregnancy. She also gives an account of the difficulties associated with maintaining secrecy in families with children conceived by gamete donation, including the particular issues raised by the practice of egg sharing.

The issue of secrecy versus disclosure from different theoretical viewpoints, together with the differing perspectives of the various parties involved, is the focus of Chapter 8 by Sharon Pettle. Based on her own interviews with people who had discovered previously unknown information about their parentage, she describes a series of stages that individuals commonly experience, from the initial revelation to integration of the new information. She then examines therapeutic approaches to working with people who have an involvement with donor conception, with particular attention to parents who wish to be open with their child and to providing therapeutic support for those who have been told about their donor conception beyond early childhood. She concludes by considering issues that are faced by therapists and counsellors who work with individuals or families with an involvement in donor conception.

In the final chapter, Ken Daniels describes the development of policy and legislation on third-party assisted reproduction around the world, with a particular emphasis on donor insemination (DI). He discusses the perspectives of the various stakeholders (DI offspring and their families, gamete providers and the medical profession), argues that public policy is essential to protect the offspring, and challenges the view that identification of gamete providers would necessarily result in a decline in donors. He also stresses the importance of national registers to enable DI offspring to access information about gamete providers. Daniels describes the situation in Sweden, where DI offspring have a legal right to identifying information about their donor, but only a minority of parents tell their children about their donor conception. He contrasts this with the situation in New Zealand where there is no legislation but only donors who are willing to be identified are recruited and parents show greater openness with their DI children. Daniels concludes with the highly significant point that a change in legislation does not necessarily lead to a change in behaviour. Instead, he argues, it is a change in attitude that is required.

In reading this collection of writings it becomes apparent that there are a number of issues that are of particular concern – notably, the question of whether or not parents of children conceived by gamete donation should be open with their children about their donor conception is addressed in all but one chapter. Most of the authors favour openness on the ground that withholding such information from donor offspring may cause psychological harm. It is also suggested that the needs of children and adults born as a result of donor conception should take priority over the wishes of parents and donors who may prefer not to tell. Nevertheless, as several authors point out, many parents decide against openness, and it is argued that parents' opinions and experiences must also be understood. Whether or not individuals conceived through gamete donation should have access to identifying information about their donor is the subject of government consultation in the UK as this book goes to press. This collection of writings will make a valuable contribution to this debate, which is likely to continue for some time.

Other important issues that recur throughout the book include selective access to infertility treatment, the implications of assisted reproduction for human rights, and conflicts between the practice of assisted human reproduction and religious beliefs. These issues all raise troublesome questions for those touched by assisted reproduction in any way. For those who are committed to tackling these controversial and difficult ethical and social issues, *Assisted Human Reproduction: Psychological and ethical dilemmas* will provide a rich and essential resource.

Professor Susan Golombok
City University, London
November 2002

Introduction

IVF blunder gives white parents black twins
Evening Standard, Sawyer (2002)

Many people's worst fears about fertility treatments seemed to have suddenly, shockingly, landed on their doorstep in the form of sensational newspaper headlines. Quickly condemned as 'an appalling tragedy' by the British Medical Association, public response was viewed as 'hysterical' by some (Birkett, 2002); while others commented that, while unfortunate, it was not a tragedy (Winston, 2002a). The regulation of legal and social parenthood in this case would take several more months to establish, and the psychological sequelae cannot be known for several more years. However, the Human Fertilisation and Embryology Authority thereafter changed its policy of 'double witnessing' which sperm fertilizes which egg and in whom the embryo is implanted, from a voluntary one to a compulsory one (Meck, 2002a). At the same time philosopher Baroness Mary Warnock, arguably the regulatory 'mother' of the infertility industry in the UK, was suggesting that her own ethical guidelines and restrictions, as set out in the 1990 Human Fertilisation and Embryology (HFE) Act were already out of date. '...The law should be changed, so that children born with the help of donors would be able to have identifying information about the donor.' (Warnock, 2002 p65). Furthermore, along with Professor Edwards the IVF pioneer, she proposed that human cloning, once proved safe, might not be psychologically or morally reprehensible (Warnock, 2002).

It seems 'we can do pretty much anything in the lab now . . . what we have to do is make sure we act judiciously in that lab' (Sauer, 2001) – a notion that strikes both hope for many couples and trepidation in others. 'Our scientific knowledge is what gives us our ethical view, and our ethics change depending on our understanding of the natural world . . . [research using "eggs" as opposed to foetuses, is ethically justified] . . . because it is designed to save, maintain and enhance human life and not destroy it'(Winston, 2002b). [For a discussion of what those involved in assisted human reproduction understand by 'eggs', see Boden et al., (2002).]

The first stem cell licences were awarded in the UK in March 2002, closely followed by the establishment of a stem cell bank, making Britain one of the most permissive countries to do so where science is regulated. The House of Lords' Science and Technology Committee, chaired by Richard Harris, the Bishop of Oxford, ruled that stem cell research on embryos was to be allowed in the UK, although this involves the use of early human life with no intent to produce a child. The Bishop was quoted as being 'satisfied on the basis of the scientific evidence that as yet research on adult stem cells has not, as some claim, made research on embryonic stem cells unnecessary' (Meek, 2002b). Despite negative reaction from religious groups, a boost in funding swiftly followed and the Human Fertilisation and Embryology Authority (henceforth the HFEA) awarded licences to two British research institutions, and the benefits thereof are predicted to come to fruition within a decade. In the USA, public funding for such research is generally tightly controlled, feeding speculation that a number of American companies might transfer some of their research activities to the UK. Both the Committee and the HFEA stressed the therapeutic purpose of these developments (aimed at curing such degenerative and chronic diseases as Alzheimer's and Parkinson's) and maintained that the regulations against human cloning remain watertight. Opinion remains deeply divided in both secular and religious communities. In the USA two of the largest groups of Orthodox Jews, representing about 1000 synagogues, expressed their support for therapeutic cloning apparently to show that there could be a moral religiously informed justification for such research [for a Jewish perspective on assisted human reproduction see Kahn, 2000].

Still under consideration in the UK are the implications of family 'sex balancing', i.e. allowing parents to choose the sex of their baby for social or religious reasons (such as, 'we already have five girls'; 'we just lost our only son'), rather than for medical reasons (e.g. to avoid sex-related hereditary or genetic diseases). Social sex selection is already available in some parts of the USA and accessible (at a price) to women of other countries. Even in the UK, for those who can afford it at a reputed cost of £8000, a trip to Belgium suffices for parents who want to choose their baby's sex (Revell, 2002).

As the technology becomes available, the use of assisted human reproduction (AHR) techniques has the potential to shift from a reactive stance of treating infertility (arguably a medical need) to an increasingly proactive stance of prenatal screening and selection to, potentially, genetic enhancement (a social want). Indeed 'the prospect of screening the entire genome at the embryo stage is not very far off' (Gosden, 1999). Consequently health professionals are finding it harder to avoid the moral and ethical issues thrown up by the advances in reproductive medicine. The need to decide how to promote the positive, but avoid or minimize the negative, consequences from the new power to alter the origins of human life is becoming more pressing.

In vitro fertilization

'The existence of IVF has made it harder for people to live with childlessness' (Leather, 2002). *In vitro* fertilization (IVF), i.e. fertilization with parents using their own gametes, raises a number of ethical questions. It is primarily available to the rich both in the UK (for a discussion of inequities of service provision in the UK, see Lord et al., 2001; Multidisciplinary Working Party, 2002) and in the USA, where only a minority of states allow fertility treatment to be included in health insurance schemes. Arguably IVF raises expectations unlikely to be fulfilled, given a success rate of 21–28 per cent between April 2000 and March 2001 (HFEA, 2002) – up from 8.6 per cent in 1986. IVF generates a surplus of embryos, the disposal of which is itself a matter of controversy and may lead to disputes in the court where partners are in disagreement. Another issue is that of multiple births where these represent 42 per cent of neonates and 70–80 per cent of pathologies (Papiernik et al., 2002). It is estimated that it costs the NHS some £60 million to treat the triplets born of IVF, on top of the financial and emotional cost to parents and the triplets themselves (Kellaway, 2002), and is often indicative of poor health outcomes. Ruth Deech, former Chair of the HFEA, contrasted these costs with the earnings of clinicians in private practice in pursuit of maximum success rates. Although not offering specific proposals, Deech (2002) suggested that some of the public cost could be borne by the private (infertility) sector. Generally the outcome seems to be that the physical health of AHR mature singleton babies is similar to naturally conceived babies (Sutcliff, 2002).

Refinements of IVF treatments have meant that sperm sorting allows embryos with desirable genes or of the desired sex to be selected for implantation, while improvements in amniocentesis tests (for an exposition, see Rapp, 1999) and the ability to screen embryos allow those predisposed to disability to be eliminated. In addition, the use of hormones in IVF treatment may increase the risk of ovarian hyperstimulation syndrome (OHSS) by 5 per cent. OHSS is a potentially life-threatening condition. It particularly affects those with endometriosis or whose infertility is the result of unknown causes (Ness et al., 2002). IVF can also lead to the paradoxical situation where a couple may be advised against unprotected intercourse during the course of ovarian stimulation (Milki et al., 2001). Those who maintain that infertility can in many cases be overcome 'naturally' have flagged concerns about what they consider to be an over-hasty resort to technological assistance or what they see as an over-emphasis on high-tech means of conception (Glenville, 2000; Barbieri et al., 2001; Payne, 2002).

Treatment is rarely confined to neat categories and, once a technology exists, its use widens. Thus, it is no longer only married couples who seek assistance. Single women, even if they have never had a sexual relationship (so-called 'virgin births'), unmarried or same sex couples, older women, postmenopausal couples (with or without children from a previous relationship), women born without a uterus, survivors of cancer or other traumatic illness who may need surrogacy, and mothers wanting to start a second family hoping to use their daughter as a known egg donor – all now have the possibility of attempting to achieve the previously unthinkable.

Lone conception

In early 2000 the HFEA permitted the use of frozen eggs in fertility treatment, directed primarily at young women suffering from illnesses such as cancer. Even before this event a commercial company called Time of Life was set up to assist single women – for a joining fee – to prepare themselves for lone conception initially using donated gametes. The options proffered are 'artificial insemination, self insemination by a known donor, and sex' (Time of Life International website). These women often prefer to remain anonymous, not admitting membership to friends or colleagues for fear of the stigma and accusations of being 'unscrupulous "sperm-hunters, . . . tampering with nature"' (Kerr, 2001). Often the stated preference was for frozen eggs, despite the low chances of pregnancy (1–2 per cent). Another company followed, originally on the Internet, as an introductory agency for lesbian and single women to male sperm donors. This led to media criticisms of indiscriminate pandering to a 'baby on demand' culture (Lockett, 2002; Brinkworth, 2002).

There are no statistics available as to how many women go forward to become mothers in this way. The social pressures to be independent career women, coupled with the demise of marriage, are often cited for the growth of this group. Others argue that media representations that it is safe to postpone the decision to have children cannot be relied on, as many women in their late 30s discover that it can be too late for them to conceive (Hewitt, 2002; Conran, 2002; Earle and Letherby, 2002). On the whole, motivation to become a parent in this way seems to be linked to the perception that time to find a partner in the usual way has run out (Murray and Golombok, 2002).

By October 2002 the first UK baby was born from the frozen egg of her genetic mother, opening the door to engineering patterns of childrearing. Dr Gillian Lockwood, who pioneered a new unfreezing technique, acknowledged that this might become 'the ultimate kind of family planning', particularly for younger women postponing parenthood to concentrate on their careers (Bosley, 2002). Is the wish to postpone parenthood unreasonable? What of the stories and individuals behind the headlines? [Names have been altered]:

> Eva, a white heterosexual English woman with retired parents, feels she has much to offer a child – love, stability and a warm family environment. At 38 she is a financially secure university graduate based in Europe. Past relationships have not worked out. Given her age she wants to store frozen embryos using her own eggs and donor sperm for future use in clinic A. Simultaneously she wants to freeze her eggs at clinic B. Should she find a suitable (and fertile) partner she plans to use her own eggs, but if this were unsuccessful she would use the embryos stored in clinic A.
>
> Were she to be a lone parent she would return home where she has a stable network of supportive friends with children. Were she not to use the embryos created on her behalf, she would donate them to other infertile couples.

Delayed birth

The number of births to women aged 45-54 rose to over 4500 in the USA in 2000, the last year for which figures are available, the highest number recorded in that age group in 30 years (Associated Press, 2002). Older and postmenopausal mothers appear to be the brunt of particular opprobrium. These women are generally discussed in the media as an 'offence' against nature, whereas older fathers may be admired or envied for their prowess (Mobiot, 2001). Findings that older male sperm have a larger number of chromosomal abnormalities do not generate the same media interest (Prestes et al., 2001). Older mothers have been criticized not in terms of their ability to parent but for being 'unnatural'. Yet, arguably, children whose parents have gone to a great deal of effort to conceive them are more likely to be loved than those conceived accidentally, and mature women are likely to have more experience and patience than younger counterparts. Late births may mean that a young child may suffer the death of his or her mother prematurely. Does this constitute sufficient reason to refuse treatment, especially as, in the developed world at least, life expectancy is greatly increased?

AHR techniques have opened the doors to intermixing relationships previously considered unalterable, raising unease about the blending of generations, potential sources of conflict with respect to 'ownership,' and possibly competing emotional claims on the resulting child(ren). The following is an example of a proposed daughter-to-mother donation:

Jane, a 40+-year-old woman who had previously been married, and Adam, her partner of over a decade, have been trying for a child together for years. After several failed fertility treatments, including advertising (unsuccessfully) for an unknown donor, Jane's adult daughter spontaneously offered to act as egg donor.

In her early 20s, she has had one five-year relationship, which has now ended. Adam has been her stepfather since she was little. Jane's first marriage was brief and her first husband offered little support.

Adam is childless. The couple live with Jane's daughter (the proposed donor) and adult son. The couple own their own business, employing the daughter and other members of their extended family. Jane's son is unaware of the proposal. The couple claim that they intend to be open with the prospective child. Should treatment be successful and there were additional embryos, the couple might try for another child.

Although Jane has tried to shield her daughter from her distress at her inability to conceive again, they have talked extensively and at times she has been unable to conceal her pain. The daughter believes that she will be unaffected by the donation – the child would be a sibling she expects to baby-sit. She wants children in the future and wants any spare eggs frozen for her own future use. Should something befall her parents, she would take on full responsibility for the prospective child.

What are the implications for the various parties if treatment proceeds? How will the family negotiate these special relationships? How should the issue of information sharing be handled? On what basis could treatment be refused?

Surrogacy

In the UK surrogacy is viewed as the treatment of last resort. It is illegal in Austria, Germany, Sweden and Norway. In Finland, Greece and Ireland surrogacy takes place with no legislative provisions. In Australia it is allowed, but not on a commercial basis. France, Denmark and the Netherlands prohibit payment to surrogate mothers. In the UK only 'reasonable' expenses are permitted. Laws vary across the USA: Arizona, New Jersey and Michigan opt for a complete ban; others such as Florida allow it with certain conditions. Those who cannot receive treatment in their own area will often seek it in other jurisdictions.

The major religions seem to be united in their opposition to surrogacy. This is based on the view that the right to reproduce means a right to have one's own children to rear. Where there is no intent or ability to rear – as in surrogacy – there is no fundamental moral right to reproduce (Steinbock, 1995). In contrast, in the secular world some advocate the advantages of openness and commercialization in the area of surrogacy (O'Driscoll, 2001). O'Driscoll cited various Hollywood stars such as

Robert De Niro, Cheryl Tiegs and Kelsey Grammer (Frasier) who had commissioned women to carry their child for them and their partner, dubbing it 'the celebrity tip of an affluent middle-class iceberg'. This is in sharp contrast to recent bans on surrogacy in China and Australia. As in the UK, US figures are largely speculative, but Shirley Zager, director of the Organization of Parents Through Surrogacy is quoted as putting the number at about 1000 annually; the UK equivalent is 415 facilitated surrogacy births since 1988. At the time of writing, California is the only American state where surrogacy agreements have legal force.

As a result of improved technological techniques, most surrogacy arrangements use the commissioning couples' gametes, which are then 'hosted' by the 'gestational carrier', avoiding a genetic link to the surrogate. Such arrangements tend to come with a price: openly in the USA, under the guise of 'reasonable expenses' in the UK where advertising for a surrogate by individuals or couples is against the law. Yet how relevant is this when seeking a surrogate seems freely available on the Internet? Anecdotally, there are reports of private surrogacy arrangements for fees in the region of £50 000, where there is no screening or contract of agreement between the parties, as promulgated by the British organization Childlessness Overcome Through Surrogacy (COTS). Is this the dreaded 'commodification' of life predicted by earlier opponents of AHR techniques, or a reasonable empowerment for those willing and able to pay an upfront fee for service? On the other hand, a recent study showed that surrogacy is often associated with good parenting (MacCallum and Golombok, 2002).

The Internet can also act as a means of anonymous communication where donor sperm can, for example, be shipped in a vial to those who request it, with no questions asked as long as payment is forthcoming. Infertile Israeli women recently won the right to import ova from abroad, meaning from Romania, apparently the greatest potential source of eggs (Siegel-Itskovich, 2002). Thus the issue of competing interests arises again and again, often couched in terms of family values versus scientific progress, rich versus poor, powerful versus powerless.

Third-party conception

Third-party reproduction raises particular psychological and ethical issues. As a medical treatment it came into its own in 1984 (the first baby conceived using donor eggs was born in 1987), and involves using the gametes (sperm or eggs) or embryos of people external to the prospective (social) family unit. Medically the need for this can arise because the male partner cannot produce sufficient or adequate quality sperm, or because the woman cannot produce eggs, e.g. the result of illness such as cancer, polycystic ovaries or a premature menopause (for a discussion of premature menopause, see Singer and Hunter, 2000).

More than 12 500 individuals have been born by donor insemination (DI) in the UK since 1991, when the HFEA was charged to keep records of all gamete transactions. There are probably another 3000 people conceived from donor eggs or embryos (Department of Health, 2001), and there may be a further 20 000 conceived before 1991; no-one knows as there was no requirement to keep records. For those born after 1991 in the UK, the earliest they will be able to access information about their gamete provider (donor) is 2008. Of course, they would need to have either been told by their parents or suspect their status in order to consider approaching the HFEA. They cannot yet be provided with identifying information about their provider. It has been argued that the information available should be increased at least to provide recipients with reassurance, and if the donor-conceived individuals are to be told, the information 'should be sufficient for them to fill in the first chapter of their life story' (Pennings, 2000).

This remains a controversial area: the climate in the UK does not appear to be ready to take up the radical notion that information regarding the means of conception be included on a donor-conceived individual's birth certificate. Yet the current situation has been criticized as too casual with calls being made for even nominal payment to (sperm) 'donors' to cease; for the quality of information gathered about them to be improved and the information verified; and for a means of updating their medical information for the benefit of their donor-conceived offspring (e.g. in the event of an inherited disease).

At their 2002 conference, the British Medical Association overturned an earlier decision of its ruling council that future people conceived from donor sperm should have the right to discover their father's identity. On the other hand, the British Fertility Society, comprising medical and allied health professionals, although against radical reforms, were urging the government to allow non-identifying information of donors to be made available, initially through a Voluntary Contact Register (Hunt and Fleming, 2002). At the same time the British Infertility Counsellors Association (BICA) strongly supported access to identifying information in the future (BICA, 2002).

Welfare of the child

What are the psychological implications for donor-conceived individuals? Could confusion and insecurity result, particularly among those who have been told that they have been conceived using donor gametes but are denied further information about their biological origin? How can the negative impact of secrets held about one's identity be assessed, or that of an unplanned discovery of such secrets? There are as yet no clear answers. In practice these issues tend to be presented as a matter of risk assessment to prospective parents. The options they are expected to consider are secrecy, partial disclosure (presented as a kind of drip-feed over time) or full disclosure from the start. Those who argue against information sharing, primarily parents and some in the medical professions, believe that donor-conceived people may find the information disturbing or alienating and that it may adversely affect their relationships with family and peers. Equally, certain religious perspectives, which do not subscribe to the virtues of AHR technology, may influence parents not to risk future ostracism of themselves or their children from their religious group. Furthermore, such information as is available is incomplete, and may be more likely to confuse or frustrate than satisfy, resulting in 'genetic bewilderment'. Weighed against this are arguments that donor-conceived individuals have an inalienable right to know their origins, and that children may be psychologically damaged if they sense an inexplicable – and conclude a shameful – difference from their social parents. The presumption is that it is better not to withhold information about origins, and that genetic information needs to be stored securely and made available so as to avoid unwitting genetic incest later on – and in future, DNA testing would quickly settle the matter.

Should there be legislation, which is notoriously slow to change, in a field driven by dazzling new possibilities at an ever-faster rate, particularly when restrictions vary from country to country, so that those who can afford it travel elsewhere for their treatment of choice? Whose rights are paramount – the adults' longing for a family at almost any cost or the prospective individual's future well-being? Can such an apparent dichotomy of interests be reconciled? Is it a matter of unadulterated consumerism primarily in individualistic, highly developed, highly technological Western cultures or, if not, on what basis can apparently competing 'rights' be regulated or adjudicated, and how and to what extent can these be enforced in practice?

For AHR is more than a series of amazing technical feats. It is at once about how human beings can be created and about how social relationships are formed – how these evolve throughout a lifetime and arguably beyond, affecting future relationship patterns and potential psychological make-up. In the past most people have appealed to 'blood ties' and the bonds of 'flesh and blood' as the basis of social obligation. Kinship ties and family life have defined how human beings make sense of the world (Finch, 1989). Until recently, a special connection between the social and the natural has been presumed, although the meaning of this may be interpreted differently across cultures. Nevertheless it constituted a recognisable given, an anchor to reality. AHR raises questions of the psychological impact of people living in families in which such traditional assumptions about kinship and family life are being challenged.

To a greater or lesser extent, part of everyone's identity as a person derives from their beliefs about their birth and upbringing. This information has necessarily involved other people and as such is also social knowledge, reaching out into how these relationships are governed and adjudicated, as in the laws of inheritance. The relationship of donor, recipient and resulting individual is exceedingly complex. The motivation of gamete providers can be complicated and this is likely to have psychological ramifications for the resulting donor-conceived person.

The meaning of these various relationships and the motivations involved are likely to have a significant impact on all concerned, e.g. does a child born using AHR techniques believe that 'their' gamete provider did so for commercial or altruistic reasons? Does the gamete provider(s) wish to have contact with the 'child', and if not what might this mean to the donor-conceived individual? At present, relatively little is known from the donor-conceived person's point of view. What psychological impact might the donor have on the family? Arguably this method of reproduction might create a triangle among the donor, the genetic parent and the non-genetic parent. This could recede into the background of everyday life but may reappear at significant junctures such as birthdays, weddings or the birth of the donor-conceived adult's own children, or it may arise in an unfamiliar fleeting gesture or a particular talent, or become a major factor in a medical history with a hereditary illness. Where only one parent is genetically related, the balance of power in the marital relationship may also be affected, as may the ease of attachment to the child.

Relationships can break down. A recent example in Scotland ruled that a gay sperm donor for a lesbian couple, who had been named on the birth certificate as the father, had visited the 18-month-old baby frequently and had contributed financially, had full parental rights, against the couple's wishes. This highlighted some of the legal difficulties faced by same sex couples that in this instance were not considered a valid family unit (Scott, 2002).

Donor-conceived individuals: the offspring

At a British Fertility Counselling Association study day, a 47-year-old man spoke of feeling excluded from his own story, of feeling 'less than fully human' and of being 'conceived by syringes'. He advocated the formation of an ethical framework for full disclosure and contact with the gamete provider (Heyworth, 2001). Christine Whipp, a 46-year-old grandmother, says that she always sensed that she did not 'fit'. When she was 40 her mother – with whom she had a difficult relationship – died, leaving a letter revealing 'that my father was a glass jar with a blob of sperm in it' . . . 'I . . . feel like a freak, a fake . . . I don't feel I know who I am any more'. Another 36-year-old woman discovered how she was created when her mother 'blurted it out' during a heart-to-heart. She questions why individuals like herself will never be able to know their genetic roots, particularly as changes in adoption were made retrospectively (Braid, 2002).

The introduction of the Human Rights Act in 1998 in the UK, which came into force in October 2000, led to almost instant challenges to the HFEA. Two actions were lodged, one in respect of sex balancing by a couple wanting to use preimplantation diagnosis to choose the sex of the embryo and a second by another couple challenging the restriction of the use of embryos. 2002 saw the first legal proceedings against an embryologist and consultant under the 1990 Act. In late 2002, the embryologist concerned was found guilty of conducting 'futile and painful operations' on women to pay off his debts (BBC, 2002). Further cases are outstanding. Most hinge around the delicate balance between the need for careful regulation and consumers' 'right' to procreate (McGleenan, 2001).

Increasingly, coverage in the media and elsewhere seems to favour the donor-conceived individual's 'right to know' in the UK and elsewhere (Dyer, 2002a, 2000b; *Rose and Another* v *Secretary of State for Health and HFEA*, 2002). One possibility currently before the Canadian parliament, which could be adopted in the UK, would allow all children conceived using donor gametes to be given full medical information about the gamete provider (but not information about his or her identity).

Even under the current arrangements half-siblings, conceived before the 1990 legislation came into force, are managing to find each other. Using DNA testing, David Gollancz (2002), who has written and spoken publicly about his feelings, has linked up to his half-brother and -sister, Barry and Janice Stevens, who were brought up in Canada. Both sets of parents were treated at a Harley Street clinic. Barry made a film called 'My Sperm Donor Dad' screened on BBC 4 in March 2002. All three believe that they may have several more half-siblings. For them, questions of nature versus nurture are lived on a daily basis (Jacobus, 2002).

As these voices begin to be heard, the notion of a register similar to that for adopted people seems to be gaining ground. Crawshaw (2002) suggests that a proportion of donor-conceived individuals will want identifying information about their gamete providers and some may also want face-to-face contact with their 'donor'. Based on recent work on adoption (Howe and Feast, 2002), she also expects that more female than male offspring will undertake searches. The two most likely single triggers for tracing are expected to be: becoming a parent and the death of a (social) parent. As in adoption, although some may want to meet their genetic parent, they may not want to establish a relationship with them. Given that these discoveries are likely to be emotionally challenging, provision may need to be made for psychological support because, as Campbell (2002) suggests, notions of the welfare of the child should be based on the concept of the child as a gift rather than a commodity.

This book

The often sensational stories described above raise complex ethical questions for individuals and for various social institutions, representing the law, the government, religious groups, clinical treatment centres, parents and offspring. Conversations with people anxious to have a child reveal their rationales and often heartfelt pleas for treatment, however unorthodox. These provide a cultural lens through which views can be explained, but essentially leave unanswered the ethical issues involved along with the long-term psychological and social implications. As more new and unusual treatments are proposed and enacted, the ground of those conducting ethical debates is constantly shifting. Media headlines and even some of the literature primarily question who should make decisions and on what basis, but there are also significant ethical and psychological issues raised by day-to-day clinical practice that affect families for a lifetime. We therefore hope that this book moves away from the sensational towards the ordinary in terms of struggling with the ethical issues and psychological consequences of AHR. By bringing together a wide range of perspectives, we hope to present a reasonably up-to-date overview of the complex dilemmas faced by the many and varied 'stakeholders' involved.

It is of course impossible to provide definitive answers or to address all the possible scenarios that might occur, but knowledge of the varied perspectives on AHR and their implications can help towards greater understanding and a more reasoned debate. The focus of the book is primarily on developments of policy and practice in the UK, particularly in respect to issues raised by third-party reproduction.

References

Associated Press (2002) Egg donation on the rise as alternative for women in their 40s and 50s seeking pregnancy. Report on www.intelihealth.org, February 13 2002, consumer health site of the Harvard Medical School.

Barbieri RL, Domar AD, Loughlin KR (2001) Six Steps to Increased Fertility. Harvard Medical School: Simon & Schuster.

BICA (2002) Executive Committee. BICA response to the Department of Health Consultation on the provision of information about donors. Journal of Fertility Counselling 9(2): 22-26.

Birkett D (2002) Why has the response to the black IVF twins born to white parents been so hysterical? The Guardian 10 July: 9.

Boden J, Hunt J, Williams DI (2002) When (and what) is an egg? Human Fertility 5(2): 47-50.

Bosley S (2002) Frozen egg baby hailed as fertility milestone. The Guardian 11 October: 11.

Braid M (2002) Your daddy was a donor. Observer 20 January: 1.

Brinkworth L (2002) Call this motherhood? Daily Mail 25 October: 34-36.

British Broadcasting Corporation (2002) Radio 4 News, 11 December.

Campbell AV (2002) Reproductive medicine: the ethical issues in the twenty-first century. Human Fertility 5(suppl): S33-S36.

Conran S (2002) Guide to Work–Life Balance 2001/2. London: Work Life Balance Trust.

Crawshaw M (2002) Donor anonymity: Lessons from a recent adoption study to identify some of the service needs of, and issues for, donor offspring wanting to know about their donors. Human Fertility 5(1): 6-12.

Deech R (2002) on 'Start the Week with Jeremy Paxman'. Radio 4, 25 March; The Times April 13, 2002.

Department of Health (2001) Donor Information Consultation: Providing information about gamete or embryo donors. London: DoH.

Dyer C (2002a) This affects thousands. The Guardian 21 May: 14.

Dyer C (2002b) Pressure increases on UK government to remove anonymity from sperm donors. British Medical Journal 324: 1237.

Earle S, Letherby G (2002) Whose choice is it anyway? Decision making, control and conception. Human Fertility 5(2): 39-41.

Finch J (1989) Family Obligations and Social Change. Cambridge: Polity Press.

Glenville M (2000) Natural Solutions to Infertility: How to increase chances of conceiving and preventing a miscarriage. London: Piatkus Books.

Gollancz D (2002) Give me my own history. The Guardian 20 May: 18.

Gosden R (1999) Designing Babies: The brave new world of reproductive technology. New York: WH Freeman.

Hewitt SA (2002) Baby Hunger. Kent: Atlantic Books.

Heyworth S (2001) Meeting Report: 2008 a turning point for truth? Counselling and legislation for the future. Human Fertility 3: 255-258.

HFEA (2002) New IVF Data, www.hfea.gov.uk, 30 August.

Howe D, Feast J (2000) Adoption, Search and Reunion: The long term experience of adopted adults. London: The Children's Society.

Hunt J, Fleming R (2002) Department of Health Information Consultation: Providing information about gamete or embryo donors. Human Fertility 5: 97-98.

Jacobus H (2002) Sperm counts. Jewish Chronicle Opinion & Features 15 March: 33.

Kahn S (2000) Reproducing Jews: A cultural account of assisted conception in Israel. Duke University Press.

Kellaway K (2002) The baby factory. The Observer 14 July: 1-2.

Kerr J (2001) Natal attraction. Time Out 11-18 July: 16-17.

Leather S (2002) quoted in 'A matter of life and death', by Bosley S, The Guardian 6 September: 6-7.

Lockett J (2002) Lesbian baby clinic opens. The Guardian 16 September: 3.

Lord J, Shaw L, Dobbs F, Acharya U (2001) Provision of fertility services: a time for change and a time for equality – infertility services and the NHS. Human Fertility 4: 256-260.

MacCullum F, Golombok S (2002) Families through Surrogacy. Human Reproduction Abstracts MS Num. V-0245 06/04/02 p1.

McGleenan T (2001) Legal issues in fertility treatment. Human Fertility 4: 270-273.

Meek J (2002a) Double witnessing to be enforced. The Guardian 5 November.

Meek J (2002b) Millions in grants for embryo stem cell research. The Guardian 28 February: 2.

Milki AA, Hinckley MD, Grumet FC, Chitkara U (2001) Concurrent IVF and spontaneous conception resulting in a quadruplet pregnancy. Human Reproduction 16: 2324-2326.

Mobiot G (2001) Our strange fear of older mothers. The Guardian 25 January: 22.

Multidisciplinary Working Party of the British Fertility Society, National Infertility Awareness Campaign and CHILD, the National Infertility Support Network: LMA Shair (Chairman), Balen H, Lenton E, Brain C and Greenwood B (2002) National Health Service provision for the management of infertility: The case for funding and reorganization of fertility services in the UK. Human Fertility 5: 167-174.

Murray C, Glombok S (2002) Going it alone: Solo mothers and their donor insemination children. Human Reproduction Abstracts MS Num. V-0524 09/04/02 p1.

Ness RB, Cramer DW, Goodman MT et al. (2002) Infertility, fertility drugs, and ovarian cancer: a pooled analysis of case-control studies. American Journal of Epidemiology 155: 217-224.

O'Driscoll E (2001) What's yours is mine. Guardian G Section 3 October: 8-9.

Papiernik E, Sage JC, Pouly JL, Mourouvin Z, de Mouzon J (2002) Multiple pregnancy outcome after assisted reproductive technology: a 25,000 deliveries Fivnat study. Human Reproduction Abstracts MS. Num V-0790 o7/04/02 p1.

Payne NB (2002) The Fertility Solution: A revolutionary mind-body process to help you conceive. London: Thorsons.

Pennings G (2000) The right to choose your donor: a step towards commercialisation or a step towards empowering the patient? Human Reproduction 15: 508-514.

Prestes EM, Sartorelli EMP, Mazzucatto LF, de Pina-Neto JM (2001) Effect of paternal age on human sperm chromosomes. Fertility and Sterility 76: 1119-1123.

Raphael DD (1981) Moral Philosophy. Oxford: Oxford University Press.

Rapp R (1999) Testing Women, Testing the Fetus: The social impact of amniocentesis in America. London: Routledge.

Revill J (2002) Parents pay to choose baby's sex. The Observer 8 September: 1, 10.

Rose and Another v Secretary of State for Health and HFEA (2002) EWHC 1593.

Sauer M (2001) IVF Scientists juggle ethics and innovation. Quoted in Ballantyne A, The Times 13 July: 10.

Sawyer P (2002) IVF blunder gives white couple black twins. Evening Standard 8 July: 1, 5.

Scott K (2002) Gay donor wins parental rights. The Guardian 8 March: 9.

Siegel-Itskovich J (2002) News roundup – Israeli women can buy ova from abroad. British Medical Journal 324: 69.

Singer D, Hunter M (2000) Premature Menopause: A multidisciplinary approach. London: Whurr.

Steinbock B (1995) A philosopher looks at assisted reproduction. Journal of Assisted Reproduction and Genetics 12: 543-551.

Sutcliff AG (2002) IVF Children: The first generation. London: Parthenon Publishing.

Warnock M (2002) Making Babies: Is there a right to have children? Oxford: Oxford University Press.

Winston R (2002a) The birth of black twins to white donors is an error, not a tragedy. The Guardian 10 July: 16.

Winston R (2002b) How would you like your egg? Update. Tel Aviv: Weizman Institute Foundation.

CHAPTER 1

Assisted human reproduction: contemporary policy and practice in the UK

ERIC BLYTH, NINA MARTIN AND CLAIRE POTTER

Implementation of the Human Fertilisation and Embryology Act 1990 (hereafter the 1990 Act) in 1991, instituting a legislative framework for the provision of assisted conception services, resulted in the UK becoming the first country in the world to establish a body, the Human Fertilisation and Embryology Authority (HFEA), with statutory powers to license and regulate centres providing assisted conception treatment.

The UK model has been portrayed as an exemplar that other countries may usefully emulate. Blank (1998, p. 148), for example, claims that: 'it has the potential for offering an optimal mixture of private input and public control if the technical aspects are derived from professional guidelines . . . . This licensing model of regulation has the advantage of public control and programme accountability that is lacking under a private, professionally controlled model.'

We have necessarily been selective in our choice of material for this chapter, which highlights key issues in the provision of, access to, and outcomes of assisted conception services that have important social, psychological and/or ethical implications and which, more than a decade since the implementation of the 1990 Act, remain problematic as a result of the legislative framework and/or regulatory system. In this chapter we consider: the development of assisted conception services and their regulation in the UK; the welfare of the child; private and NHS assisted conception services; infertility counselling; surrogacy arrangements; consent and posthumous conception; payment to donors; access to information about genetic origins after third-party assisted conception; and the role of the HFEA in licensing and regulation.

Assisted conception procedures

A number of assisted conception procedures are discussed in this chapter. Below is a brief description of these:

- Gamete intrafallopian transfer (GIFT) is a procedure that involves ovarian stimulation, egg retrieval and the transfer of the eggs and sperm into the fallopian tube. If fertilization occurs, it does so *in vivo*.
- *In vitro* fertilization (IVF) is the fertilization of an egg outside the body, usually in a petri dish, using either 'donor' sperm or the sperm of the partner of the recipient woman, hence the term *in vitro* and the vernacular usage 'test tube'. The egg(s) is/are extracted by transvaginal ultrasound guided retrieval, usually under local anaesthesia and may also be accompanied by a pharmaceutical regime to encourage superovulation and the production of more eggs. The embryo(s) is/are then transferred to the uterus. In addition to using the gametes of the woman who is receiving treatment, IVF can also be used in conjunction with 'donated' eggs or embryos.
- Intracytoplasmic sperm injection (ICSI) is a procedure involving the injection of a single sperm into an egg. This is a technique that enables a man with few sperm to become a genetic father. Once an embryo has been created, this is transferred to the uterus as in IVF.
- Posthumous conception describes the use of a deceased individual's gametes or embryo for the purposes of assisted conception.
- Genetic surrogacy is a surrogacy arrangement in which the eggs of the surrogate mother (the woman carrying the pregnancy) have been used to create the child. Consequently, the surrogate mother is both the birth mother and the genetic mother of the child. Conception will usually have been achieved following insemination of the commissioning father's sperm. It is also known as 'straight', 'partial', or 'genetic-gestational' surrogacy.
- Gestational surrogacy is a surrogacy arrangement where the surrogate mother has no genetic relationship to the child she is carrying. Conception will usually have been achieved following IVF using the oocytes and sperm of the commissioning parents. Also knows as 'IVF', 'full' or 'host' surrogacy.

Finally we comment on use of terminology such as 'donor' and 'donation'. Daniels (1998) convincingly challenges the unqualified use of such terms since, in practice, very few 'donors' actually 'donate' their gametes or embryos without some measure of financial gain or reward in kind. Although we have retained use of 'donor', 'donation' and similar terminology, such as 'donor-conceived' people, not only to ensure consistency with existing literature and research, but also because of a failure to devise sufficiently succinct alternatives that command common acceptance, the reader should be aware of this caveat.

The development of a regulatory framework in the UK

The regulatory framework in the UK owes its provenance to the Warnock Committee, appointed by the Government in July 1982:

> to consider recent and potential developments in medicine and science related to human fertilization and embryology; to consider what policies and safeguards should be applied, including consideration of the social, ethical and legal implications of these developments; and to make recommendations.
>
> DHSS (1984, p. 4)

Although the Government responded to Warnock (DHSS, 1984) with a relatively protracted consultation (DHSS, 1986, 1987) before implementation of the 1990 Act in 1991, the medical profession speedily established a voluntary regulatory body, initially called the Voluntary Licensing Authority (subsequently the Interim Licensing Authority) which was in operation by 1985. Thus, it might be argued that UK medical practitioners embraced early on the concept of the regulation of assisted conception. An alternative interpretation is that the medical profession realized the inevitability of regulation and that, if it took the initiative, it would be well positioned to influence the development and control of services and research. In the event this is substantially what did happen and although, subsequently, concerns were expressed about the impact of legislation and regulation, the response of the medical and other relevant professions towards regulation has been generally positive (see, for example, Brinsden, 1993; Lieberman et al., 1994; Winston, 1999; for a dissenting view, see Edwards, 1998). Indeed, over two-thirds of 'persons responsible' for licensed assisted conception units, who responded to Lieberman and colleagues' survey investigating the operation of the 1990 Act, were in favour of gamete intrafallopian transfer (GIFT), formally outwith the Act's regulatory provisions, being brought within the regulatory framework on the grounds that its exclusion 'perpetuates an inferior standard of care for many infertile couples while exposing the woman to the same risks as IVF' (Lieberman et al., 1994, p. 1781). In practice, most GIFT treatment in the UK is provided by licensed centres and is therefore subject to the Act's regulatory provisions (HFEA, 1995, p. 21).

The 1990 Act permits the provision of a wide range of assisted conception treatments, including sperm, egg and embryo 'donation', IVF, GIFT – and variations, intracytoplasmic sperm injection (ICSI), posthumous conception, and both genetic and gestational surrogacy. Other forms of assisted conception treatment, such as the prescription of fertility-enhancing medication that has potentially important implications both for the welfare of individuals and for the commitment of public resources, are totally disregarded by the 1990 Act (Bennett and Harris, 1999). Included among the relatively few prohibitions are certain commercial activities associated with surrogacy, while the HFEA prohibits use of preimplantation genetic diagnosis for 'sex selection' other than for 'genuine' medical reasons. Any ambiguity regarding restrictions on cloning has been resolved in the courts. In November 2001, in a case brought by the ProLife Alliance, the High Court ruled that cloning by cell nuclear replacement (CNR) fell outside the remit of the Human Fertilisation and Embryology Act. The government appealed this decision and also fast-tracked legislation prohibiting the transfer of a cloned embryo into a woman. The Human Reproductive Cloning Act, however, forbids the implantation of cloned embryos only, not their creation. The government also indicated that it would introduce measures to regulate the cloning of human embryos for therapeutic purposes. In January 2002, the Court of Appeal reversed the High Court decision, determining that the spirit of the Human Fertilisation and Embryology Act had been to include cloning by CNR. At the time of writing, the ProLife Alliance is reported to be considering an appeal to the House of Lords (Rumbelow, 2002).

Few formal limitations are imposed on access to treatment, the major factor limiting eligibility being that treatment must not be provided to a woman 'unless account has been taken of the welfare of any child who may be born as a result of the treatment (including the need of that child for a father), and of any other child who may be affected by the birth' (Section 13(5)). An associated requirement, which we explore further below, is that treatment must not be provided unless 'proper counselling' is offered to the woman and to any partner she may have (Section 13(6)). Provisions for counselling availability also apply to prospective donors (Section 3(3)(1)(a)) and to individuals born as a result of donor-assisted conception who seek information about their genetic origins (Section 31(3)(b)). Where donated genetic material is provided, the Act generally protects the anonymity of the donor, although it makes provision for donor-conceived people to obtain some information about their genetic heritage (Section 31). We discuss this in more detail below.

The HFEA is required to:

- regulate, license and monitor centres that offer treatment using donated gametes, or involving the creation of human embryos outside the body, store human gametes or embryos, or carry out research on human embryos
- maintain a Register of Information about donors of gametes and embryos used for the treatment of others, recipients of such treatment and children born from those treatments, and arranging for access to information held on the Register in accordance with the law
- produce and maintain a Code of Practice, giving guidance about the conduct of licensed activities
- publicize its role and provide relevant advice and information to patients and donors and to clinics
- 'keep under review information about embryos and any subsequent development of embryos and about the provision of treatment services governed by the Act and to advise the Secretary of State, if he asks it to do so, about those matters' (Human Fertilisation and Embryology Act, 1990 Section 8(a))
- produce an annual report to Parliament.

The first chairman of the HFEA, Sir Colin Campbell, observed that the Authority had two over-riding priorities: 'that the interests of all those involved are recognised by properly informed and thorough analysis of the issues and that people seeking treatment and donors should receive the highest possible standards of service' (Campbell, 1993).

What needs to be noted, however, is that the HFEA is responsible for a relatively limited range of assisted conception services; Winston (1999, p. 151) commented that: 'the HFEA has no control over the great bulk of reproductive medicine'.

Access to assisted conception services

The welfare of the child

The principal legislative criterion concerning treatment eligibility is the welfare of the child requirement. Although at face value this might appear both necessary and laudable (as it must have appeared to legislators), its operationalization has been fraught with difficulty, as we indicate below.

Such problems appear to have been expected by the Warnock Committee (Warnock, 1987), although the Committee's report itself is surprisingly mute on these. Indeed, the Committee's failure to articulate these difficulties, and to alert well-meaning legislators to them, has at least a part to play in the implementation of legislation strong on rhetoric, but in which symbolism and good intentions would exercise primacy over consequences. In the event, unambiguous commitment to the welfare of children was not the sole motivation for legislators, Section 13(5) owing more to Government compromise in the face of the endeavours of right-wing MPs trying to prevent treatment being provided to single women and lesbians (Blyth, 1995a).

The British Fertility Society's (1999) conclusions that 'A definition of the meaning of "welfare of the child" has not yet been agreed and in its absence, implementing the assessment is, in practice, the subject of confusion and debate' have been endorsed by other commentators on the operationalization of the Act (see, for example, Douglas, 1993; Lieberman et al., 1994; Blyth, 1995a; Blyth and Cameron, 1998; Patel and Johnson, 1998; Harris, 2000; Langdridge, 2000).

The framework for considering the welfare of the child in both the HFEA Code of Practice (HFEA, 2001a, 3.13–3.15) and the British Fertility Society's *Recommendations for Good Practice – welfare of the child* (BFS, 1999), which focus on parenting competence and the suitability of potential treatment recipients to rear children, gives credence to Tizzard's (1999) critique of 'talk of child welfare [as] really a smokescreen for the more unpalatable reality of weeding out unfit parents', marital status and sexual orientation providing a major basis for the determination of 'unfitness' (see Douglas, 1993; Englert, 1994; Deech, 2002).

Several key limitations flow from this narrow interpretation of welfare. First, little encouragement is given to consideration of the welfare of the individual beyond his or her childhood or to broader or longer-term issues. These include self-identity and the importance of knowledge about one's genetic origins, either for the promotion of a positive self-image or for the benefit of one's own descendants (and which, we argue below, is compromised in the case of donor-conceived individuals by the limitations placed on the availability of information about their genetic heritage). Second, as Leese and Whittall (2001, p. 172) observe, it would be reasonable to infer that welfare should also encompass the 'notion of "health" in a biological sense' – another aspect of welfare that, to date, has received little attention. Third, the Act does not afford the welfare of the child any priority; it merely requires that account be taken of it, but mandates no further action. In addition, the requirement to take into account the welfare of 'any other child who may be affected by the birth' simply adds to the range of potentially competing interests, including those of existing children, children who do not yet exist and prospective parents, influencing decision-making within treatment centres.

Private and NHS health care in assisted conception

In its gatekeeping role, the welfare requirement interacts with financial considerations. Since 1993, the National Infertility Awareness Campaign (NIAC) has commissioned six surveys on funding and provision of assisted conception services in the UK (College of Health, 1993; Wiles and Gordon, 1994; Wiles and Patel, 1995; Wiles and Oddos, 1996; Stone and Reisel, 1997; Kennelly and Reisel, 1998). These have identified considerable regional variability in both the level and the range of publicly funded assisted conception services, e.g. some local NHS funding bodies have decided not to fund assisted conception treatment at all, whereas others apply strict eligibility criteria relating to the age, sexual orientation and marital status of applicants. Limited funding for treatment results in waiting lists of varying duration. Funding bodies are not bound by the provisions of the 1990 Act, although they are required to comply with the Human Rights Act 1998. Given Brown's (2000, p. 268) observation that 'subfertility treatment on the NHS is not just rationed: it is patently arbitrary and totally unethical', NHS provision for assisted conception services may find itself tested against the rights guaranteed under the Human Rights Act. For the present, however, upwards of 75 per cent of people seeking assisted conception services fund their treatment themselves (Kerr et al., 1999; Deech, undated), thus circumventing NHS waiting lists and eligibility criteria.

Our final observation here is to note the differences in eligibility criteria imposed by treatment centres providing NHS funded services and those providing private treatment. Centres providing NHS treatment are more likely than their private counterparts to operate a rationing policy and impose more restrictive eligibility criteria because of the limited availability of NHS treatment and the need to demonstrate accountability for the deployment of public resources. In contrast, as a result of the relative freedom of manoeuvre offered by the 1990 Act and the HFEA's 'light-touch' approach to practice in individual centres (see below), private centres may provide treatment to whomsoever they choose with virtual impunity (Brazier, 1999; Bennett and Harris, 2001; Levitt, 2001; Rogers, 2001).

Infertility counselling

At first sight, the decision to include consideration of counselling in a debate focused on access to treatment might seem questionable, if not perverse. However, we believe that the origins of infertility counselling and current debates about its practice justify its inclusion here.

The foundations for the provision of infertility counselling in the UK were laid by the Warnock Committee, which recommended that 'non-directional' counselling 'should be available to all infertile couples and third parties at any stage of the treatment' (DHSS, 1984, para. 3.4, p. 16). The Committee's recommendations were largely incorporated within the 1990 Act, requiring that 'proper counselling' be made available to people considering treatment, those intending to be donors and to donor-conceived individuals seeking information about their genetic origins from the HFEA Register of Information.

Before implementation of the 1990 Act, it was formally acknowledged that much counselling in infertility treatment centres was focused on treatment failure, and was provided by medical and nursing staff who not only possessed no specialist counselling training, but were also responsible for providing the (failed) treatment (Voluntary Licensing Authority, 1986; Frew, 1989). The Government clearly saw counselling as having a measure of independence from medical care. It: 'should be distinct from discussions with a doctor of any medical treatment he [*sic*] proposes and should be carried out by somebody different, preferably a qualified counsellor' (DHSS, 1987, para 77, p. 13).

Given that infertility counselling was not a developed specialty, the Department of Health commissioned the King's Fund Centre to assist the HFEA in defining the nature and role of 'proper counselling' in licensed treatment centres (King's Fund Centre, 1991). The HFEA accommodated a number – but by no means all – of the King's Fund Centre recommendations and incorporated these in its Code of Practice (HFEA, 2001a). (For a discussion of the development of infertility counselling in the UK, see Blyth and Hunt, 1994.)

In addition to making suggestions about the nature, content and role of infertility counselling in licensed treatment centres, the King's Fund Centre recommended that all centres should employ at least one person trained in infertility counselling and that a training programme should be instituted to ensure necessary expertise. The HFEA imposed less stringent demands, requiring licensed centres (other than those engaged in research only) to ensure: 'either that at least one of its staff has a Certificate of Qualification in Social Work or an equivalent qualification recognised by the Central Council for Education and Training in Social Work, or is accredited by the British Association of Counsellors, or is a Chartered Psychologist, *or that a person with such a qualification is available as an advisor* to counselling staff and as a counsellor to clients as required' (HFEA, 1993, para. 1.10, p. 5 – our emphasis).

The King's Fund Centre proposed a time-frame for the introduction of specialized training, although in the event its modest targets were not achieved, and only in October 2001 did specialist training and accreditation for infertility counsellors come on stream. Although this programme produced the 'first fully accredited infertility counsellors in the world' (Monach, 2001, p. 7), resource limitations have imposed significant restrictions on the pace of development of accreditation and, over a decade after implementation of the 1990 Act, only a handful of infertility counsellors who, in the opinion of relevant professional bodies, possess the necessary experience and qualifications will be offering a service in the UK. There is no timescale to ensure nationwide provision. In recognition of the new accreditation programme, the HFEA modified its qualification requirements for counsellors in its most recently revised Code of Practice (HFEA, 2001a, para 1.10, p. 10), although in practice this still means that a suitably qualified counsellor, as defined by the HFEA, may never actually see a patient or a donor, because they need only to be 'available'.

Despite continuing promotion of the 'non-directive' model for counselling (HFEA, 1991), Section 13(5) meant that some mechanism had to be developed to enable the child's welfare to be taken into account. The Government White Paper, *Human Fertilisation and Embryology: A framework for legislation* (DHSS, 1987, para 78, p. 13), linked counselling with assessment for eligibility to treatment, albeit ambiguously and, during parliamentary passage of the Human Fertilisation and Embryology Bill, the Government identified the potential role of counsellors in 'dissuading' some people from proceeding with treatment (Mackay, 1990). The King's Fund Centre (1991, p. 13) saw a clear role for counselling and the protection of the child's interests:

> In our view it will be impossible to separate the process of counselling from consideration of the welfare of the child.

Although the King's Fund Centre provided a mandate for counsellors to be involved in welfare assessments, Douglas (1993, p. 67) underscores their competence to do so: 'trained counsellors may well be more likely than the medical team to have the skills and knowledge to carry out a welfare assessment, and more likely to obtain a real understanding of the patient than the doctor could do in a fairly brief consultation'.

Despite its efforts to maintain a distinction between counselling and the process of assessing prospective treatment recipients or donors (HFEA, 2001a, para 8.2, p. 36), the Code of Practice advises: 'the views of all those at the centre who have been involved with the prospective parents should be taken into account when deciding whether or not to offer treatment' (HFEA, 2001a, para. 3.25, p. 18).

In practice, the tension between providing 'independent' and 'non-directional' counselling, membership of the centre's multidisciplinary team and the need to take account of the welfare of the child continues to exercise practitioners. Counsellors themselves are ambivalent about their role in assessment (Blyth and Hunt, 1994; Williams and Irving, 1998). However, research studies have identified both the development of *de facto* compulsory counselling, especially for certain social groups, such as single women and lesbians, or for people seeking certain types of treatment, such as donor conception, egg sharing and surrogacy, as an integral element of a centre's assessment processes and the difficulty of making welfare assessments (Douglas and Young, 1992; Blyth, 1995a; Blyth, 2001a). Finally, empirical evidence indicates low levels of patient uptake of counselling (Hernon et al., 1995; Boivin et al., 1999; Kerr et al., 1999). When so few patients access counselling, we must question how far it can be seen 'as part of normal routine' (HFEA, 2001a, 8.5, p. 36).

Surrogacy arrangements

The origin of difficulties surrounding the legislative framework governing surrogacy arrangements derives from division within the Warnock Committee; most of the Committee wished to see surrogacy prohibited, although two dissenting members perceived surrogacy as an option of last resort, but which, because of the complex issues it raised, should be closely regulated. This dissension was not resolved during the pre-legislative consultation process and, although the government accepted the 'last resort' argument, it seemed to take the view that regulation would afford surrogacy some legitimacy and so decided not to include it within the proposed regulatory framework. The 1990 Act was, therefore, intended merely to tighten up existing legislation, the Surrogacy Arrangements Act 1985, which had itself been hurriedly implemented in the wake of the 'Baby Cotton' case (Cotton and Winn, 1985; Blyth, 1993a), re-emphasizing that surrogacy arrangements would not be enforceable in British courts, and clarifying ambiguity left by the 1985 Act about parental relationships after a surrogacy arrangement. The 1990 Act confirmed the status of the child's birth mother in a surrogacy arrangement as the child's legal mother in both gestational and genetic surrogacy, i.e. regardless of whether or not she was also the child's genetic mother (Section 27). Determination of the child's legal mother also had implications for determination of the child's legal father (Section 28). Depending on the birth mother's marital status and the precise nature of the surrogacy arrangement, the child's legal father could be the surrogate mother's husband, the 'commissioning' father (if he was the child's genetic father), a sperm donor (if he was the child's genetic father) or no one at all (Blyth, 1995b).

While the Human Fertilisation and Embryology Bill was being debated in Parliament, a case of genetic surrogacy (which at that time was still relatively infrequent) received a high level of publicity and was instrumental in the introduction of what is now Section 30 of the Act – albeit without the benefit of extra-parliamentary discussion or much parliamentary debate – initiating a new measure, the parental order; this order enabled a married couple to assume parental responsibility for a child born as a result of a surrogacy arrangement (Blyth, 1993b). Conditions under which a parental order may be sought after the birth of a child through a surrogacy arrangement are set out in Section 30 of the Act. The conditions that need to be met are that:

- at least one of the applicants requesting the order must be a genetic parent of the child
- at the time of the application and the making of the order, the child's home must be with the applicants
- the application must be made within six months of the child's birth (special transitional arrangements were made for applications in respect of children born before the implementation of Section 30)
- at the time of the application and the making of the order, both applicants must be domiciled in the UK, the Channel Islands or the Isle of Man
- at the time of the making of the order, both applicants must have attained the age of 18
- the court must be satisfied that both the child's legal mother and legal father give their informed consent freely and unconditionally to the making of the order. Such consent cannot be dispensed with (e.g. on the grounds that it is being 'unreasonably' withheld – as in adoption proceedings). However, the agreement of the father or the mother is not required if they cannot be found or are incapable of giving their agreement. This is a particularly important point if the child has no legal father
- the child's mother cannot give her consent less than six weeks after the child's birth
- the court must be satisfied that the birth mother has received no money or other benefit (other than for expenses reasonably incurred) from the applicants in connection with the application or relinquishing care of the child to them, unless authorised by the court.

Implementation of Section 30 proved problematic and was not achieved until 1 November 1994, the Minister of Health, Tim Sackville, conceding that the provisions were 'considerably more complex than they first appeared' (Sackville, 1994). Arguably, the complexity of the proposals and the future legislative problems inherent within them might have been more apparent had they been subject to adequate levels of public, professional and parliamentary scrutiny at the time.

Despite evidence of the increasing acceptance of surrogacy in the UK and the establishment of one of the most liberal regimes for surrogacy within Europe (Blyth, 1998), emerging concerns about certain aspects of its practice prompted a Government review (Brazier et al., 1998). Although the team appointed to undertake the review judged that 'across a wide spectrum of opinion . . . the existence of surrogacy is now accepted, and that the crucial issue is how far the state should intervene to protect the interests of the parties' (p. 30), it also reported that 'the incomplete implementation of the recommendations of either the majority or the minority of the Warnock Committee [has] created a policy vacuum within which surrogacy has developed in a haphazard fashion' (p. i). The review team was concerned that the inadequate scrutiny of 'reasonable expenses' permitted under Section 30 had effectively led to the development of a commercial market in surrogacy, and recommended both increased restrictions over the payment of expenses and the establishment of a new regulatory framework representing a policy of 'containment' (Brazier, 1999, p. 183). Although the Government proposed further consultation on the review team's recommendations, at the time of writing nothing further has been heard about the Government's intentions, and the practice of surrogacy in the UK remains substantially unchanged.

Consent and posthumous conception

Problems over the Act's consent provisions for the storage and use of an individual's gametes emerged in the highly publicized case of Diane Blood (1997, 2001). Mrs Blood's husband, Steven, was suddenly taken fatally ill with meningitis in 1995. At the time the couple were actively trying for a family, although not by means of assisted conception. While Mr Blood was still alive, although comatose and unlikely to recover, Mrs Blood persuaded a doctor to take some sperm from him by means of electro-ejaculation so that she could use this to achieve a pregnancy. Subsequently Mr Blood died without regaining consciousness. Crucially, he had not consented to the storage of his sperm, as required under the provisions of the 1990 Act (Section 4(1)(b)), and the HFEA refused permission for Mrs Blood to be treated with his sperm (although she was, of course, eligible to request donor insemination using the sperm of an anonymous donor who might also have died since donating his sperm). Mrs Blood initiated legal action to get the treatment she wanted and eventually the Court of Appeal ruled in her favour, because it considered the

HFEA to be in breach of the Treaty of Rome (Articles 49 and 50) which allows a citizen of an EU member state to receive medical treatment in another member state. Mrs Blood was given permission to 'export' her husband's sperm to Belgium (*R v Human Fertilisation and Embryology Authority ex parte Blood*, 1997), where she was successfully treated and her son, Liam, was born in December 1998. Following the Blood case the Government commissioned a review of the Act's consent provisions (McLean, 1998). In July 2002 Mrs Blood gave birth to a second posthumously conceived son.

McLean concluded that the existing requirement for written consent was appropriate, given the range and complexity of the decisions to which consent of this nature applies. However, she recommended the introduction of a 'best interests' test to permit the removal and storage of gametes of an individual who is not competent to give his or her consent, pending their decision once competence is achieved or restored. Where any doubt exists about the likelihood of the individual's recovery or the impact of treatment on the individual's fertility, a court should determine the lawfulness of the proposed removal. Where a court has declared that it is in the 'best interests' of a person who is not able to give consent to have gametes removed, the HFEA should have the power to waive the consent requirements for storage. The Government initiated a further consultation exercise on Professor McLean's recommendations. However, as with the surrogacy review, there is no further news of a timescale for any action.

The Blood case raised another key issue. As Mrs Blood was a single woman at the time of her insemination, in accordance with Section 28 of the Act, her son Liam has no legal father, although the identity of his genetic father is not in doubt. McLean recommended amendment to Section 28(6) so that, in cases similar to those of the Blood family, the child's genetic father would be given legal recognition. Although the Government appeared sympathetic to the Blood family – and to the 30 or so other families in a similar situation – this did not extend to making available Government time to permit the necessary change in legislation, and consequently a private member's Bill (the Human Fertilisation and Embryology [Deceased Fathers] Bill 2001), sponsored by Labour backbench MP Tony Clarke, sought to secure this. Although the Bill received cross-party support, it was talked out of time by Conservative MP, Desmond Swayne, on its third reading in the House of Commons, becoming a casualty of the dissolution of Parliament in advance of the 2001 general election. Personal communication with the Department of Health since the re-election of the Labour party indicates that new proposals are planned to give effect to the intentions of the Deceased Fathers Bill, although at the time of writing there are no firm proposals for bringing forward any legislative change.

Payment to donors

Payment to donors may be made only if authorised by means of directions issued by the HFEA (Section 12(e)). When the Authority was established, as sperm donors had customarily been paid, it allowed existing centres to continue to pay donors a maximum of £15. However, the Authority made clear its objection to payment 'in principle as it risked the quality of the consent that was given and was inconsistent with the view that gamete donation should be a gift, freely and voluntarily given' (Deech, 1998, p. 82).

The Authority instituted a consultation process to determine the best way of phasing out payment (HFEA, 1998a). However, in the face of clinician-led opposition, in December 1998 the HFEA abandoned its proposed withdrawal of payment, a decision that unambiguously showed that ethical values had been trumped by practical considerations:

> It has become clear from the responses to the recent consultation that the removal of payment in the present climate would seriously jeopardise the supply of sperm donors . . . . We therefore feel it is important that the supply of safe, cryopreserved sperm in the UK remains adequate and do not feel that £15 payment is so wrong that we were prepared to threaten the entire service.
>
> Deech (1998b)

At the same time, the Authority directed that centres established since 1991, which had hitherto been prevented from making any payment at all, would also be allowed to pay donors up to £15. The HFEA gave no indication then, or subsequently, about how it intended to pursue its professed continuing commitment to the withdrawal of payment.

Arrangements for the remuneration of egg donors has been, and remains, somewhat different – globally its practice representing the extremes of the altruism–commercialism spectrum in assisted conception. In the UK, egg donation has generally been characterised by altruism, as noted by Winston: 'Woman regard [egg donation] largely as an altruistic act giving the pleasure and fulfilment of a child to another individual' (Winston, 1999, pp. 152–153).

Altruistic donation is closely aligned to the position taken by the Council of Europe that: 'the human body and its parts shall not, as such, give rise to financial gain' (Council of Europe, 1996, Article 21, Chapter VII).

An International Consensus on Assisted Procreation, drawn up by the International Federation of Fertility Societies, an association of 50 professional bodies, states 'there should be no compensation to . . . donors for providing the oocytes. However, this does not exclude the reimbursment [*sic*] for expenses, time and risk which are associated with the donation' (International Federation of Fertility Societies, 2001). Nevertheless, commercial egg 'donation' is prevalent, especially in the USA, where egg 'donors' may be hired via a commercial agency for a fee ranging up to $US15 000. [See, for example, the website for Fertility Alternatives Inc. (www.geocities.com/fertilityalternatives/oocyte.html) which offers the services of 'intelligent' and 'exceptional' donors – most of whom are university students. In communities where there are shortages, e.g. among Jewish and African–American individuals, the fees proffered can be substantial. The Ethical Committee of the American Society for Reproductive Medicine has stated that reasonable financial inducements are justified given the time, pain and effort (and potential health risks) involved, but these should not discriminate against lower income women or be exploitative (ASRM, 2000).]

However, in the UK, quite apart from disquiet about the ethics of remunerating sperm donors while expecting egg donors not only to undergo a far more invasive procedure, but to do so altruistically, concerns began to emerge about the potential risks of donating posed to women not otherwise undergoing their own fertility treatment (Ahuja and Simons, 1998). In response to this, and the associated problems of a shortage of donor eggs, a long waiting list for treatment with donor eggs and the limited availability of publicly funded assisted conception treatment, Ahuja and his colleagues (2000) pioneered the system of 'egg sharing' – a means of offering 'free' or subsidised IVF treatment to women willing to donate eggs for the treatment of others. The HFEA started from a position of undisguised antipathy towards egg sharing, having described it as an 'unacceptable' practice (HFEA, undated) that should be 'phased out' (Johnson, 1997). However, responses to the consultation on the withdrawal of payment to donors provided evidence of more ambivalent attitudes towards egg sharing than those expressed by the HFEA itself (Blyth, 2001b), and the Authority decided that egg sharing should be 'regulated, not banned' (HFEA, 1998b) – although this should not been taken as indicating that the HFEA had given egg sharing its 'ethical approval' (HFEA, 1999a). In October 2000, the Authority issued *Guidance for Egg Sharing Arrangements* (HFEA, 2000), which has since been incorporated in the fifth edition of the HFEA Code of Practice (HFEA, 2001a).

The key issues in egg sharing, in addition to those generally associated with the use of donated gametes identified by the HFEA, include the possible conflict of interest between the donor and recipient, especially where the same centre is providing treatment to both parties, and also recognition of the donor as a patient. To ensure that the interests of both donors and recipients are adequately safeguarded, the HFEA requires centres to make available to both parties an individual, 'such as a nurse', to provide 'impartial support' throughout the process. The individual providing support for the donor should be different from the person providing support for the egg recipient(s). The provision of such 'impartial support' appears to be seen by the HFEA as different from the provision of counselling, although this is not made explicit. With regard to counselling, the HFEA recommends that 'all couples' contemplating participation in egg sharing should receive implications counselling – the possibility that either a donor or recipient might not be in a relationship appears not to have crossed the minds of the authors of the guidance. In practice, most assisted conception treatment centres providing egg sharing have instituted mandatory counselling (Blyth, 2001a). The HFEA further requires centres to make explicit the minimum number of eggs that need to be available for the egg sharing arrangement to proceed, the arrangements for allocating eggs between the donor and recipient(s), and details of costs. The agreement should make clear that, if the minimum number of eggs needed for sharing are not produced, the egg donor should be given the option of using all her eggs at no additional cost to her and with no further commitment.

The HFEA also appears to have used this opportunity to extend restrictions on the provision of information in donor-assisted conception contained in the Act, by advising centres that donors and recipients should not be told the outcome of each other's treatment (HFEA, 2001a, Annexe A, (v) (b), pp. 55–56). At the same time, the Authority has charged counsellors with the responsibility of dealing with the implications of this policy, in particular the implications of not knowing whether treatment for the other 'couple' has succeeded or not, and the implications of the possibility that any child born after treatment might have one or more half-sibling(s) of a similar age (HFEA, 2001a, p. 40). For a more detailed critique, see Blyth (2001b).

Access to genetic origins information in third-party assisted conception

Competing claims, on the one hand to privacy by donors and recipients of donated gametes or embryos and, on the other, to information about their genetic origins by donor-conceived individuals have posed a particularly persistent dilemma, not only in the UK, but also in many parts of the world (see, for example, Shenfield and Steele, 1997; Blyth, 1998; Frith, 2001; McWhinnie, 2001). Although the Warnock Committee was not convinced of the merits of donor-conceived individuals being able to learn the identity of the donor, it did recommend that when a donor-conceived individual reached the age of 18 he or she 'should have access to the basic information about the donor's ethnic origin and genetic health' (DHSS,

1984, para 4.21, pp. 24–25). However, the Committee did not consider that such provisions should have retroactive effect.

The Act essentially follows the recommendations of the Warnock Committee, generally safeguarding the donor's anonymity. Currently, the only circumstances under which the identity of the donor may be revealed are by order of a court in the 'interests of justice' or in connection with any legal proceedings that may be initiated as a result of a child being born with a congenital disability (Human Fertilisation and Embryology Act 1990, Sections 34–35), while providing access to certain information where the applicant has been given a 'suitable' opportunity for counselling.

To reduce the risks of consanguinity, Section 31 of the Act permits an individual intending to marry (i.e. from the age of 16) to ascertain whether the HFEA Register of Information provides any evidence of a genetic relationship to his or her intended spouse (given the nature of twenty-first century personal relationships, a somewhat anachronistic device that is likely to have limited effect). At the age of 18 an individual may ask the HFEA whether he or she was born as a result of licensed treatment including that using a donated embryo or gametes.

The Act also allows the Government to make Regulations specifying any additional information held on the Register that may be disclosed to a donor-conceived individual on reaching the age of 18. Although this information could include the donor's identity, retroactive disclosure of donor identity by means of Regulations is specifically prohibited. In December 2001, the Department of Health (2001a) issued a consultation document to assist decision-making on what information – if any – should be made available to donor-conceived individuals. However, the failure hitherto of the Government itself to issue regulations, and therefore pre-scribe the nature of information to be included on the Register, has created a policy vacuum that the HFEA has tried to address.

Initially, the HFEA obtained information from centres about donors on the Donor Information Form (HFEA Register (91) 4), which required details about the donor's height, weight, ethnic group, eye colour, hair colour, skin colour, occupation and interests, and whether the donor has any children of her or his own. This form also included a small space for donors to provide 'a brief description' of themselves that could be given to recipients and to any child subsequently born. More recently, this form has been superseded by Donor Information Form (99) D.1.0 which is similar in many ways to the earlier form, except that this no longer asks for information about the donor's height or weight, but does enquire about the donor's religion. The Authority advises centres to encourage donors: 'to provide as much . . . non-identifying biographical information about themselves as they wish, to be made available to prospective parents and any resulting child' (HFEA 2001a, 4.4, p. 20).

On the Authority's own admission, the welfare of people conceived after donor treatment was not the main priority in determining the nature of information about donors sought by the HFEA. Rather it was perceived as: 'the *minimum necessary* to allow the Authority to answer questions from children born as a consequence of treatment services about their genetic backgrounds . . . . Great importance was given in the design of the data collection system to avoid *unnecessary intrusion* into the personal lives of patients and donors, and to avoid *unnecessary cost* to centres and to the Authority (HFEA, 1992, p. 23 – our emphasis).

It is not clear on what basis the Authority determined what would constitute either 'necessary' or 'unnecessary' in this context, and the HFEA's approach to the collection of donor information needs to be contrasted with its requirement on centres that: 'the degree of consideration [regarding the welfare of the child] necessary will be greater if the treatment is required to be licensed under the HFE Act and *particularly if it involves the use of donated gametes*' (HFEA, 2001a, para. 3.9, p. 16 – our emphasis).

In consequence, the quality of the information collected by the HFEA, and which will provide the basis of any information that may subsequently be released to donor-conceived individuals, is variable (Maclean and Maclean, 1996; Abdalla et al., 1998; Blyth and Hunt, 1998) and, whatever any future regulations may determine, they will offer little benefit to donor-conceived individuals who have already been born.

Provisions for donor-conceived individuals to access genetic origins information stand in contrast to arrangements for an individual born as a result of a surrogacy arrangement and subject to a parental order, who has a right to access her or his original birth record and thus discover the identity of her or his surrogate mother. However, the effect of different legal systems within the UK has created a further anomaly, in that in Scotland this information can be accessed from age 16, but in the remainder of the UK not until the individual has reached the age of 18. It is also likely that an applicant in Scotland may be able to access more information than applicants elsewhere in the UK (Douglas et al., 1998).

In advance of any action that may be taken by the Department of Health on the basis of response to its consultation, the English High Court took a major step in July 2002, in the case of Joanna Rose, a 29-year-old donor-conceived woman, and an unidentified six-year-old girl, who claimed that statutory enforcement of donor anonymity in the UK contravened their right to 'respect for private and family life' guaranteed by Article 8 of the 1950 European Convention (*Rose and Another v Secretary of State for Health and Human Fertilisation and Embryology Authority*, 2002). In light of the Department of Health Consultation, the Court adjourned until the consultation had concluded. Nevertheless the judge, Mr Justice Scott Baker, was clear that the applicants' request to obtain information about their biological fathers 'goes to the very heart of their identity' and was an essential element of 'private life' protected by the European Convention. The judge added:

> It is to my mind entirely understandable that AID children [*sic*] should wish to know about their origins and in particular to learn what they can about their biological father or, in the case of egg donation, their biological mother. ... an AID child [*sic*] is entitled to establish a picture of his identity as much as anyone else' (*Rose and Another v Secretary of State for Health and Human Fertilisation and Embryology Authority*, 2002).

In October 2002, the UN Committee on the Rights of the Child added to this debate in its report on progress on implementation of the UN Convention on the Rights of the Child in the UK, expressing concern that donor-conceived people have no right to know the identity of their biological parents (BBC, 2002b).

The HFEA: licensing and regulation

The final area on which we wish to comment concerns the relationship between the HFEA and licensed treatment centres. The 1990 Act outlines the HFEA's statutory licensing and regulatory role, giving it authority to withdraw, or refusal to renew, a centre's licence. Less drastically, the HFEA may impose conditions on a licence. However, the 1990 Act is not the sole determinant of the nature of the HFEA's relationship with treatment centres. The Government has placed the HFEA in a symbiotic relationship with centres by determining that, in order to restrict the demands made on the public purse, 70 per cent of the HFEA's costs should be met through licence fees. The government has maintained pressure on the HFEA to seek an increasing share of its revenue from clinics and in 2002, the Authority issued proposals on how an additional £4 million required to ensure the necessary delivery of services could be met from revisions to the licence fee structure (HFEA, 2002a).

The potential compromise of the HFEA's independence from the centres it regulates is emphasised by the constitution of the Authority's part-time inspectorate, most of whom are themselves employed in treatment centres. Therefore, not only is the relationship between inspector and inspected mediated by personal and professional familiarity, but the roles are frequently interchangeable. Winston (1999, p. 149) has accused inspection teams of a 'serious lack of uniformity and objectivity', although his proposed remedy – the establishment of a professional inspectorate – did not find favour with the HFEA itself (HFEA, 1999b). In addition, although there are statutory limitations to the representation of providers of assisted conception services on the HFEA itself, a significant proportion of HFEA members are service providers. Given this context, the espousal

by the Authority of a 'light touch' in its dealings, both with individual centres and in terms of its overall relationship with centres, is not particularly
surprising: 'The [HFEA] guidelines define expected practice, but they are
framed in a way which allows clinicians to make different decisions in individual cases where these can be justified' (Deech, 1998, p. 83).

> [The HFEA] does not, in general, work prescriptively by imposing its own
> procedures and practices but works by asking clinics to develop and justify
> theirs within the law in order to grant a licence.
>   Patel and Johnson (1998, p. 769)

As we have illustrated above in our review of the operation of the 1990
Act, significant issues in which the HFEA has a margin of discretion, such
as the policy on payment to donors and arrangements for collecting information from centres about donors, have been 'resolved' in ways that suit
the interests of service providers, even where the outcome may be at odds
with declared ethical principles.

The relationship between the Authority and centres may also help
explain the lack of transparency of decision-making, especially with
regard to centre inspections. In its early years, the HFEA used its annual
reports to provide summary information about the outcomes of the
licensing process for the previous year and investigation of alleged
breaches of the Code of Practice. However, the 1996 Annual Report
(HFEA, 1996) was the last to provide any information about the issue of
licences with conditions, and the 1997 Annual Report (HFEA, 1997) was
the last to make any reference to investigation of alleged breaches of the
Code of Practice. It has also become apparent that not even members of
inspection teams see the final report relating to any inspection in which
they have participated, that is prepared by the HFEA's Licence Committee.
The lack of transparency in the inspection process was the subject of
adverse comment in the latest quinquennial review of the HFEA (DoH,
2001b), which appears to have had some impact in that the HFEA has
recently agreed to make public – on request – both inspection reports and
minutes of the Licence Committee minutes (HFEA, 2001b).

Conclusion

At the outset of this chapter we cited Robert Blank as an enthusiast of the
UK model of regulation. However, he also warns that: 'legislation . . . risks
freezing technology in place and is unlikely to offer the flexibility needed
to adapt to new applications' (Blank, 1998, p. 135).

Brinsden, advocating a 'better-the-devil-you-know' approach, concedes
that: 'Some clinicians and scientists are concerned that more and yet

more regulation of their practices will occur, and yet there is at present no more qualified body to consider these matters. Surely better that this Authority, with its greater depth of knowledge and experience than any other, should be tasked with debating these problems, rather than some new imposed Authority of lesser experience' (Brinsden, 1993, p. 499).

Others have been less acquiescent. MP David Alton (1996), now Lord Alton, has accused the HFEA of behaving 'in an arrogant and unaccountable manner, arrogating powers to itself . . . so much for freedom of information, public disclosure or access'. Robert Edwards (1998) acknowledges the need for some legislation, but argues that this must be used 'sparingly' and should not be the primary regulatory tool because it can be both inflexible and difficult to change. Moreover, he claims that politicians, administrators and lawyers possess insufficient technical knowledge to legislate effectively, and that professional service providers should be given increased ethical authority. He envisages an 'appropriate professional organisation', such as the General Medical Council (GMC), being given this responsibility. Sadly for Edwards' proposition, the singular failure of the GMC to protect the public from the murderous predilections of family doctor Harold Shipman has effectively rendered such an option highly improbable. MPs added their weight to criticisms of the HFEA when, in July 2002, the House of Commons Science and Technology Committee questioned the HFEA's decision to allow a couple to use preimplantation genetic testing to select an embryo that could provide human tissue to help their seriously-ill son (House of Commons, 2002). The Committee claimed that the HFEA had exceeded its powers, asserting that: 'democracy is not served by unelected quangos taking decisions on behalf of parliament' (BBC, 2002a). In response, the then recently-appointed chief executive of the HFEA, Maureen Dalziel, indicated that 'new, clearer legislation is desperately needed' (HFEA, 2002b).

Given that no other acceptable options for regulation present themselves and that, in our view, there is no case for reducing regulation, we accept not only that the UK's current regulatory system will continue in more or less recognisable form for the foreseeable future, but that, in principle, this system generally offers the best way forward. However, effective regulation demands that a distinction be made between the general and relatively timeless principles that require encapsulation in legislation, and the more fluid policy and practice issues that can best be left to subsidiary regulations or to a Code of Practice issued by a regulatory body, and those issues that do not need to be regulated at all but are perhaps best left to professional body codes of practice and ethics.

The UK's experience shows that shortcomings in underlying legislation necessarily compromise the role and functioning of any regulatory body and service providers. Examples from our review above include the problems in implementing Section 30, the legalistic fudge over surrogacy arrangements, the ambiguity concerning the welfare of the child requirement and the anomalies following use of gametes from a deceased person. A further example that we have not discussed earlier arose from early realization that the original confidentiality requirements in the Act (Section 33 (5)) were excessively restrictive and, indeed, posed a threat to patient care. They prevented any person to whom a licence applies from giving information about a patient that would identify the patient to any other person not covered by a licence, save in a few clearly defined circumstances. This prevented centres from giving information about a patient, even with the patient's consent. This was a deficiency that was resolved in July 1992 when the Human Fertilisation and Embryology (Disclosure of Information Act) 1992 became law, relaxing some of the restrictions on the provision of patient information. However, the continued existence of other anomalies highlights the problems associated with deficient legislation.

In contrast to the practical difficulty of amending legislation, the HFEA has, since 1991, been able to revise its Code of Practice on four occasions and, even though the most recent edition was published only in March 2001, further revision is already being planned. However, we have also shown the limitations of a regulatory body which has struggled to meet the demands and expectations placed upon it. Given the tremendous changes that have taken place since implementation of the Human Fertilisation and Embryology Act in 1991, the time is right for a radical overhaul of the UK's regulatory system.

Table of cases

R v Human Fertilisation and Embryology Authority ex parte Blood (1997) 2 All ER (England Reports) 687, Court of Appeal
Rose and Another v Secretary of State for Health and Human Fertilisation and Embryology Authority (2002) EWHC 1593

References

Abdalla H, Shenfield F, Latarche E (1998) Statutory information for the children born of oocyte donation in the UK: What will they be told in 2008? Human Reproduction 13: 1106–1109.
Ahuja K, Simons E (1998) Cancer of the colon in an egg donor: ethical and policy repercussions for donor recruitment. Human Reproduction 13: 227–231.
Ahuja K, Simons E, Rimington M et al. (2000) One hundred and three concurrent IVF successes for donors and recipients who shared eggs: ethical and practical

benefits of egg sharing to society. Reproductive BioMedicine Online 1: 101–105.

Alton D (1996) House of Commons Official Report (Hansard) 30 October, col. 592–596.

American Society for Reproductive Medicine, Ethics Committee (2000) Financial incentives in recruitment of oocyte donors. Fertility and Sterility 74: 216–220.

Bennett R, Harris J (1999) Restoring natural function: access to infertility treatment using donated gametes. Human Infertility 2: 18–21.

Bennett R, Harris J (2001) The Welfare of the Child and access to infertility treatment. Journal of Fertility Counselling 8(3): 24–29.

Blank R (1998) Regulation of donor insemination. In: Daniels K, Haimes E (eds), Donor Insemination: Social sciences perspectives. Cambridge: Cambridge University Press.

Blood D (1997) Speech given at Westminster School, London, 26 February. Journal of Fertility Counselling 4(2): 9–12.

Blood D (2001) A personal account. Journal of Fertility Counselling 8(2): 28–31.

Blyth E (1993a) Children's welfare, surrogacy and social work. British Journal of Social Work 23: 259–275.

Blyth E (1993b) Section 30: the acceptable face of surrogacy? Journal of Social Welfare and Family Law 4: 248–260.

Blyth E (1995a) The United Kingdom's Human Fertilisation and Embryology Act 1990 and the welfare of the child: a critique. International Journal of Children's Rights 3(3/4): 417–438.

Blyth E (1995b) Assisted conception and surrogacy: the development of services. In: Richards J (ed), Surrogacy: A Guide for Guardians *ad litem* in Applications under S 30 of the Human Fertilisation and Embryology Act 1990. Liverpool University: Centre for the Study of the Child and the Family and the Law.

Blyth E (1998) Donor assisted conception and donor offspring rights to genetic origins information. International Journal of Children's Rights 6: 237–253.

Blyth E (2001a) Subsidized IVF: The Development of 'Egg Sharing' in the United Kingdom, paper given at 16th World Congress on Fertility and Sterility, Melbourne, 26 November.

Blyth E (2001b) Guidance for egg sharing arrangements: redefining the limits of information-giving in donor assisted conception. Reproductive BioMedicine Online 3(1): 45–47.

Blyth E, Cameron C (1998) The welfare of the child: an emerging issue in the regulation of assisted conception. Human Reproduction 13: 2339–2342.

Blyth E, Hunt J (1994) A history of infertility counselling in the United Kingdom. In: Jennings S (ed.) Infertility Counselling. Oxford: Basil Blackwell.

Blyth E, Hunt J (1998) Sharing genetic origins information in donor assisted conception: views from licensed centres on HFEA Donor Information Form (91) 4. Human Reproduction 13: 3274–3277.

Boivin J, Scanlan LC, Walker SM (1999) Why are infertile patients not using psychosocial counselling? Human Reproduction 14: 1384–1391.

Brazier M (1999) Regulating the reproduction business? Medical Law Review 7: 166–193.

Brazier M, Golombok S, Campbell A (1998) Surrogacy: Review for Health Ministers of Current Arrangements for Payments and Regulation: Report of the Review Team. Cmnd 4068. London: The Stationery Office.

Brinsden P (1993) The effect of the Human Fertilisation and Embryology Act 1990 upon the practice of assisted reproduction techniques in the United Kingdom. Journal of Assisted Reproduction and Genetics 10: 493–499.

British Broadcasting Corporation (2002a) 'Designer baby' ruling condemned, http://news.bbc.co.uk/1/hi/health/2134314.stm accessed 27 September 2002.

British Broadcasting Corporation (2002b) http://news.bbc.co.uk/2/hi/uk_news/politics/2300207.stm accessed 4 October 2002.

British Fertility Society (1999) Recommendations for good practice – welfare of the child. Human Fertility 2(2): 85.

Brown CJ (2000) Rationing fertility services in the NHS: the patients' viewpoint. Human Fertility 3: 268–270.

Campbell C (1993) Foreword. Human Fertilisation and Embryology Authority Annual Report. London: HFEA.

College of Health (1993) Report of the National Survey of the Funding and Provision of Infertility Services. London: College of Health.

Cotton K, Winn D (1985) Baby Cotton: For love and money. London: Dorling Kindersley.

Council of Europe (1996) Convention for the Protection of Human Rights and Dignity of the Human Being with Regard to the Application of Biology and Medicine. Strasbourg: Council of Europe.

Daniels KR (1998) The semen providers. In: Daniels K, Haimes E (eds), Donor Insemination: Social sciences perspectives. Cambridge: Cambridge University Press.

Deech R (1998a) Legal and ethical responsibilities of gamete banks. Human Reproduction 13(suppl 2): 80–83.

Deech R (1998b) Payments for egg and sperm donors. Unpublished letter. 9 December.

Deech R (undated) ART and the Family: Risk or revival, http://familycenter.byu.edu/marriageconf/media/deech.pdf accessed 18 March 2002.

Department of Health (2001a) Donor Information Consultation: Providing Information about Gamete or Embryo Donors. London: Department of Health.

Department of Health (2001b) Human Fertilisation and Embryology Authority: Quinquennial Review. London: Department of Health.

Department of Health and Social Security (1984) Report of the Committee of Inquiry into Human Fertilisation and Embryology (The Warnock Report). Cmnd 9414. London: DHSS.

Department of Health and Social Security (1986) Legislation on Human Infertility Services and embryo research. Cmnd 46. London: HMSO.

Department of Health and Social Security (1987) Human Fertilisation and Embryology: A Framework for Legislation. Cmnd 259. London: HMSO.

Douglas G (1993) Assisted reproduction and the welfare of the child. In: Freeman M, Hepple B (eds), Current Legal Problems. Oxford: Oxford University Press.

Douglas G, Young C (1992) Findings from a Survey of Issue Members. Unpublished paper. Cardiff: Cardiff Law School, University of Wales.

Douglas G, Lavery R, Plumtree A (1998) Truth and the child: the legal perspective. In: Blyth E, Crawshaw M, Speirs J (eds), Truth and the Child 10 Years On: Information exchange in donor assisted conception. Birmingham: British Association of Social Workers.

Edwards R (1998) Introduction and development of IVF and its ethical regulation. In: Hildt E, Mieth D (eds), In Vitro Fertilisation in the 1990s: Towards a medical, social and ethical evaluation. Aldershot: Ashgate.

Englert Y (1994) Artificial insemination of single women with donor semen. Artificial insemination with donor insemination: particular requests. Human Reproduction 9: 1969–1977.

Frew J (1989) Counselling in IVF Clinics: statement on behalf of the Interim Licensing Authority. The British Infertility Counselling Association Newsletter 2(autumn): 4–5.

Frith L (2001) Gamete donation and anonymity: the ethical and legal debate. Human Reproduction 16: 818–824.

Harris J (2000) The welfare of the child. Health Care Analysis 8: 27–34.

Hernon M, Harris CP, Elstein M, Russell CA, Seif MW (1995) Review of the organized support network for infertility patients in licensed units in the UK. Human Reproduction 10: 960–964.

House of Commons (2002) Developments in human genetics and embryology. Report of Science and Technology Committee. London: House of Commons.

Human Fertilisation and Embryology Authority (1991) Code of Practice: Explanation. London: HFEA.

Human Fertilisation and Embryology Authority (1992) Annual Report. London: HFEA.

Human Fertilisation and Embryology Authority (1993) Code of Practice, 2nd edn. London: HFEA.

Human Fertilisation and Embryology Authority (1995) Fourth Annual Report. London: HFEA.

Human Fertilisation and Embryology Authority (1996) Fifth Annual Report. London: HFEA.

Human Fertilisation and Embryology Authority (1997) Sixth Annual Report. London: HFEA.

Human Fertilisation and Embryology Authority (1998a) Consultation on the Implementation of Withdrawal of Payments to Donors. London: HFEA.

Human Fertilisation and Embryology Authority (1998b) Paid Egg Sharing to be Regulated not Banned. (Press release.) 10 December. London: HFEA.

Human Fertilisation and Embryology Authority (1999a) Notes of meeting of the Authority, July (www.hfea.gov.uk/frame.htm).

Human Fertilisation and Embryology Authority (1999b) Notes of meeting of the Authority, October (www.hfea.gov.uk/frame.htm).

Human Fertilisation and Embryology Authority (2000) Guidance for Egg Sharing Arrangements. London: HFEA.

Human Fertilisation and Embryology Authority (2001a) Code of Practice, 5th edn. London: HFEA.

Human Fertilisation and Embryology Authority (2001b) Minutes of meeting of the Authority, 22 March (www.hfea.gov.uk/frame.htm).

Human Fertilisation and Embryology Authority (2002a) HFEA Consultation on the Modernisation of Regulation and New Fee Strategy. London: HFEA.

Human Fertilisation and Embryology Authority (2002b) Response to the House of Commons Science and Technology Committee Report, Developments in human genetics and embryology. Press release. London: HFEA.

Human Fertilisation and Embryology Authority (undated) Working Group on the Effects of Removing Payment to Donors Policy Statement on Payment for Gametes. London: HFEA.

International Federation of Fertility Societies (2001) International Consensus on Assisted Procreation. Montpellier: International Federation of Fertility Societies.

Johnson M (1997) Payments to gamete donors: position of the Human Fertilisation and Embryology Authority. Human Reproduction 12: 1839–1846.

Kennelly C, Reisel J (1998) Report of the Sixth National Survey of the Funding and Provision of Infertility Services. London: College of Health.

Kerr J, Balen A, Brown C (1999) The experiences of couples in the United Kingdom who have had infertility treatment – the results of a survey performed in 1997. Human Reproduction 14: 934–938.

King's Fund Centre (1991) Counselling for Regulated Infertility Treatments: The report of the Counselling Committee. London: King's Fund Centre.

Langdridge D (2000) The welfare of the child: problems of indeterminacy and deontology. Human Reproduction 15: 101–103.

Leese H, Whittall H (2001) Regulation of the transition from research to clinical practice in human assisted conception. Human Fertility 4: 172–176.

Levitt M (2001) 'Not so wrong that we are prepared to threaten the entire service' – The Regulation of Reproductive Technologies in the UK. Human Reproduction and Genetic Ethics 7(2): 45–51.

Lieberman B, Matson P, Hamer F (1994) The UK Human Fertilisation and Embryology Act 1990 – how well is it working? Human Reproduction 9: 1779–1782.

Mackay Lord (1990) Official Report. House of Lords. 6 March, col. 1098.

McLean S (1998) Review of the Common Law Provisions Relating to the Removal of Gametes and of the Consent Provisions in the Human Fertilisation and Embryology Act 1990. London: Department of Health.

Maclean S, Maclean M (1996) Keeping secrets in assisted reproduction – the tension between donor anonymity and the need of the child for information. Child and Family Law Quarterly 8: 243–251.

McWhinnie A (2001) Should offspring from donated gametes continue to be denied knowledge of their origins and antecedents? Human Reproduction 16: 807–817.

Monach J (2001) The BICA/BFS Counselling Award: BICA/BFS Counselling Accreditation Project. Journal of Fertility Counselling 8(2): 7–8.

Patel JC, Johnson M (1998) A survey of the effectiveness of the assessment of the welfare of the child in UK in vitro fertilization units. Human Reproduction 13: 766–770.

Rogers L (2001) Woman to have brother's IVF child. Sunday Times 26 August: 1–2.

Rumbelow H (2002) Court of Appeal closes loophole on human cloning. The Times 19 January: 16.

Sackville T (1994) House of Commons Official Report, Vol. 248, col. 974, 26 October.

Shenfield F, Steele SJ (1997) What are the effects of anonymity and secrecy on the welfare of the child in gamete donation? Human Reproduction 12: 392–395.

Stone V, Reisel J (1997) Report of the Fifth National Survey of the Funding and Provision of Infertility Services. London: College of Health.

Tizzard J (1999) The welfare of adults. Progress in Reproduction 3(1): 3.

Voluntary Licensing Authority for Human In Vitro Fertilisation and Embryology (1986) The first report of the Voluntary Licensing Authority for Human In Vitro Fertilisation and Embryology. London: Medical Research Council and Royal College of Obstetricians and Gynaecologists.

Warnock M (1987) Ethics, decision-making and social policy. Community Care 685: 18–23.

Wiles R, Gordon C (1994) Report of the Second National Survey of the Funding and Provision of Infertility Services. London: College of Health.

Wiles R, Oddos C (1996) Report of the Fourth National Survey of the Funding and Provision of Infertility Services. London: College of Health.

Wiles R, Patel H (1995) Report of the Third National Survey of the Funding and Provision of Infertility Services. London: College of Health.

Williams D, Irving J (1998) Counselling is not assessment. Journal of Fertility Counselling 5(1): 13–15.

Winston R (1999) The IVF Revolution: The definitive guide to assisted reproductive techniques. London: Vermillion.

CHAPTER 2

Issues of gamete donation and sex selection: a clinician's view

FRANÇOISE SHENFIELD

Many issues in assisted human reproduction raise ethical dilemmas, and the choice in this chapter is necessarily eclectic. The chosen themes are gamete donation and sex selection, but one must mention other issues relevant to care in general, in particular access to treatments and the issue of justice. The restricted access to *in vitro* fertilization (IVF) treatment by post code, with its double-pronged iniquity (Shenfield and Steele, 1997) is especially relevant to couples who would try intracytoplasmic sperm injection (ICSI) if it were subsidized because of severe male oligospermia, but choose donor insemination (DI) because it is either cheaper or accessible in the NHS. More recently, issues such as those of cloning and the therapeutic hopes of stem cells, and specifically embryonic stem cells, as well as the complex choices to be made in the use of preimplantation genetic diagnosis (Pennings and Liebaers, 2002), have been making the headlines and are mentioned elsewhere (Shenfield, 2002).

Gamete donation

Certain issues surrounding gamete donation are also of relevance at the moment, especially with regard to the mostly European tradition of anonymity of the gamete donor. This must be put in the context of the identity of the offspring in relation to his or her intended (or psycho-social) parents and to his or her origins.

The fact that sperm donation has been used for many years means that we have more evidence about the follow-up of these children than we have for the offspring of oocyte (or embryo) donation; both latter techniques require the use of IVF. Studies have been published about the parents, some offspring and the gamete donors. Before detailing the relevant information, however, mention must be made of the issue of payment, or compensation, of the donors.

It seems obvious, at least from a semantic point of view (Shenfield, 1994), that a gift should be free. Indeed, the fact is that, if society intends to pay gamete donors, the term 'donation' itself should be changed to 'sale' of gametes and embryos. However, in most countries where gamete donation is used as a means of solving infertility problems, those who recruit the donors have difficulties matching supply to demand, especially in the case of oocytes. Thus, it has been argued that pragmatism should prevail in a scarce supply environment, and that some type of financial inducement should certainly not be forbidden. In the UK this, of course, must be within the frame of British law, which states that 'no money or other kind of benefit shall be given or received in respect of any supply of gametes or embryos unless authorised by directions' (Human Fertilisation and Embryology [HFE] Act 1990). The notion of making a gift is also enshrined in law in France and Spain (IFFS, 2001).

With the conviction that the human body and its parts and products should remain outside commerce, one can attempt a rational argument in the realm of ethics, in order to outline the theoretical basis to the proposition. It is based mainly on the notion of respect of the person. Without entering the very complex debate of what is the meaning of 'personhood', the special quality of respect due to the person was most cogently articulated over 200 years ago by Immanuel Kant. It stems from the observance of the second categorical imperative, 'to treat all humanity always at the same time as an end and never merely as a means' and is the symbol of the rational mind: that 'all reasonable creatures respect a human being' (Seve, 1994). The relevance of altruism to the future child, who may well be informed of his or her origins, is also important.

The utilitarian stance has sometimes been portrayed thus: in a scarce supply environment, should one choose to pay donors, can the negative consequences identified by Titmuss (1971) about the payment for blood donation be overcome? These negative consequences (to be contrasted with the obvious positive side effect of probable increase and ease of supply, for instance) centred around three main points: the discouragement of voluntary supply, the increased risk of transmitting disease by donors motivated by gain only and willing to falsify information, and potential exploitation of the weakest socioeconomic groups of society (Rodriguez del Pozo, 1994). If one replaces the word 'blood' by 'gametes', the arguments stands: paid gamete donors might falsify information and, at best, increase the cost of the recipient system when they would eventually be rejected by the thorough and appropriate screening in force; at worst, the 'welfare of the child' might be compromised by an adverse factor which would have escaped the screening. However, in view of the stringent screening put in place by the Human Fertilisation and Embryology Authority (HFEA) Code of Practice, the exploitation argument is probably the most powerful of the three Titmuss arguments.

Exploitation can have many guises, and one is coercion, even if subtle. Considering the social context in which donation is approved, as a gesture of solidarity and altruism, we wonder why these values seem to have very little meaning to Golombok and Cook's sample of prospective male donors (HFEA, 1994). The relevant finding to this article is that 'all (sperm) donors believed they should be paid and 62% reported they would not donate sperm if not paid'. The picture was different among potential female donors who 'were motivated by a wish to help rather than payment'. Sex differences have been reported before (Schover et al., 1992), but it still leaves one wondering about the psychosocial environment, which prevents donors from contemplating voluntary donation. One relevant bias introduced by the present system may be that potential sperm donors know that it has been usual, in the UK, to give limited payment in exchange for donation, a custom that then takes on a normative value. One also wonders about the effect on 'future generations' who might be aware that a commercial transaction, rather than an act of generosity, was partly responsible for their origin. Another complex dilemma is that of egg sharing. Within the European context, this is actually the only allowed method of oocyte donation in Denmark. The HFE Act 1990 allowed benefits 'for female donors' (those allowed being treatment services and sterilization), and the debate can thus be summed up as: Is this a form of coercion to donate, a form of payment or an acceptable 'exchange'?

Two different cases must be analysed: (1) 'exchange' of ova for treatment unrelated to fertility therapy and (2) exchange among women (or couples) all requiring fertility treatment:

1. The separation principle has been most eloquently put in the Polkinghorne report (HMSO, 1989) on foetal tissue. This principle, with appropriate counselling, is powerfully convincing when a woman makes the final decision of sterilization, which should be available, if or when necessary, as are other means of contraception. One can envisage women not making a fully informed decision, if they are not well counselled and given an opportunity to obtain early private treatment for which, on the NHS, there may be a long waiting list.
2. Donation of ova as part of an IVF treatment cycle is arguably easier to contemplate, because both the potential donor and the recipient are suffering from the same complaint, infertility, and the exchange between the parties seems more balanced. They are also more likely to be well informed, as are many of the patients who have been through the sometimes difficult path of fertility treatments, and for whom IVF

(and related treatments) is often the last chance of achieving a long awaited pregnancy. Thus, consent is much more likely to be informed in such cases.

The problem is nevertheless complex. It is of course compounded by the fact that both IVF and ovum donation are mostly available privately in the UK, at a cost that many potential patients cannot even contemplate. How can one ensure lack of coercion for a woman (and her partner) who gives ova in exchange for x cycles of IVF treatments, which she and her partner could not otherwise afford?

In either case, this exchange in treatment cycles is compounding the injustice of a system to which access is given on the grounds of means and not of need. While awaiting the long overdue change in access to assisted human reproduction (AHR) techniques, pragmatism has prevailed in the UK, allowing egg sharing. The latest Code of Practice (HFEA, 2001) includes a particular section on how to implement a fair approach to both donors and recipients.

First, general advice is given, stating that 'the treatment offered should be the most suitable to suit the medical needs of both the egg provider and the egg recipient', and in practice this means that 'both . . . should have access to an individual, such as a nurse, who should be available to provide impartial support'. More detailed advice also includes the usual information giving, in order to obtain informed consent, plus the 'alternative treatment available'. Of course, one alternative to egg sharing is not to share. It may be argued that it is not a therapeutic option, but, if one considers that the egg sharer may compromise her success rates by not having frozen embryos, for instance, it may indeed be part of the therapeutic option in a large sense. We await evidence from units practising egg sharing in order to assess and better inform couples considering the practice: it may be that the success rate is not compromised because a fertile donor (e.g. young, with polycystic ovaries and a male problem) has a very good chance for herself anyway. Therefore, an even harsher dilemma involves a potential egg sharer who is refused because she is too old or has a prejudiced ovarian reserve, especially if she finds the cost of the procedure difficult to bear. This is yet another argument in the realm of justice, and challenges equitable access for all couples to AHR techniques. Limits may indeed be given, but in a fair way applying to all couples, with arguments referring to the welfare of the child, the joint age of the two partners in the couple, as well as their health, thus enabling the child to have a fair chance of having at least one surviving parent till maturity (Pennings, 2001).

It goes without saying that the counselling in such cases is even more complex, time-consuming and essential. The Code of Practice stresses that implication counselling 'must . . . cover . . . the implications of not knowing whether the recipient has succeeded or not, if the provider remains childless, the implications for the recipient of using a sub-fertile egg provider, and . . . of there possibly being half siblings (to the donor's offspring of a similar age resulting from treatment)'. This has direct implications for the other topical dilemma in the field of gamete donation – anonymity and secrecy (Shenfield and Steele, 1997).

There is also wide variation in attitudes to anonymity in gamete donation in Europe, with the contrasting examples of Sweden and France which respectively enshrine known donors and anonymity in their legislation. It is therefore appropriate to ask the current question, which has been thrashed out both in medical journals and sometimes, to much publicity and with some misapprehension, in the daily press as well as other media. Should policy reverse the traditional anonymity in (especially) sperm and oocyte donation, and make access to donor identity compulsory for future children, as Sweden did in 1985 (Gottlieb et al., 2000), as is practised in New Zealand and as the Netherlands are about to do? And is this a matter of human rights?

Although starting from a position of doubt in the face of these legal challenges, it is morally essential to be one's own fiercest critic and challenge what one wrote a few years ago (Shenfield and Steele, 1997): 'anonymity has a role in the social and psychological construct of the family resulting from gamete donation, especially enhancing the social paternal role of the male in the recipient couple in case of sperm donation. Its other function is to protect privacy, as it allows a couple to keep the "artificial" means of conception of their child a secret if they so wish. This ought to be respected, as there is no evidence that it is deleterious to the child. New studies concerning children who have been told of their origins will offer evidence on the lack of secrecy of the procedure of gamete donation, but we may have to wait a long time before being able to observe the effects of known donation on children. The question is the meaning of knowing one's origins, a matter of importance to each and every one of us . . . and . . . which has . . . a varied significance, historically, psychologically and anthropologically'.

There are indeed several models for this special area of gamete donation. The Swedish and the Dutch models are well known; they are based on a similar stance, because the planned modification in the Netherlands is impending and will end the 'two-gate' system which enabled parents to choose either a donor who would undertake to disclose his identity later or one who would not, and donors themselves would also choose whether or not to make this undertaking.

In UK legislation, with the Code of Practice of the HFEA we have the following guidance: 'where people seek licensed treatment using donated gametes, a child's potential need to know about his or her origins . . . should be considered'. It is important to notice the phrasing, because there are legal nuances between a 'must' representing the necessity of hard law and a 'should'. But, we have all heard the powerful voices of anger and distress of some children of sperm donation (Gollancz, 2001), who argue that they have been deprived of specific knowledge, the identity of the genetic sperm provider (avoiding the legal and emotional term 'father'), information without which they do not find their sense of identity complete. However, one very important caveat is that in most cases the interests of children and parents seem to coincide because several studies have already shown that children conceived by 'assisted reproduction' fare very well on the measured personal and social criteria, when compared with children conceived 'naturally' or adopted (Golombok et al., 1996).

It is, however, extremely difficult to gather evidence on the subject, as we know that secrecy was maintained by most prospective parents who chose DI for conception of their child in a European study. The psychoanalytical approach to secrecy in family relationships is a relevant factor to take into consideration as well (Weil, 1992), although we all, both privately and socially, have specific attitudes about anonymity in gamete donation that are shaped by our culture and sometimes our prejudices, rather than by evidence.

One may therefore attempt to gather and compare the available evidence, even though others have argued that most of the available psychosocial studies in the field of disclosure of information suffer from serious methodological flaws, prohibiting any firm conclusion (Broderick et al., 1995). Finally, a contextual approach is also needed, especially within the arguments often used about 'knowing the truth for a child is a Human Right' in our post-modern world.

Our theme is enlightened by the Dutch and Swedish experience to date. Part of the basis for the Swedish stance stems from arguments in favour of 'the right of the child' to know of his or her 'origins', and the potentially divisive role of secrets in families. When one enters the area of rights and finds a conflict of interests between those claiming rights, it is difficult to ascertain which might take precedence. In this particular case, do we, for instance, prioritize the 'right to privacy' of the parents and donors, or the 'right to know' of the prospective child? The first right is actually inscribed in the European Convention on Human Rights, recently integrated in UK legislation (Human Rights Act 1998). Indeed Article 8 entails the right to respect for private and family life, home and correspondence. The second is enshrined in the International Declaration of Children's Rights and alludes to the right of children to know their family, which again begs interpretation.

At this stage, it is necessary to define what is a right, or at least a negative right:

> . . . in most cases when we say that someone has a 'right' to do something,
> we imply that it would be wrong to interfere with his doing it, or at least
> that some special grounds are needed for justifying any interference.
>
> Dworkin (1991)

These very special grounds are indeed stated in the European
Convention for Human Rights 1950. Taking into account the fact that
Article 8 may underline a conflict of interests between the privacy interests of parents and donors, and other interests claimed by the offspring,
one may try to obtain further knowledge from evidence published, while
at the same time taking into account a new approach, by Pennings
(2001), describing the right to know one's origins as a positive right, but
specifically included in the right to privacy.

The evidence on secrecy and anonymity has been gathered from the
parents. In 1995, Cook and colleagues studied 45 families with a child
conceived by DI, compared with 55 families with an adopted child and
41 with a child conceived by IVF. The children were between ages 4 and
8 at the time and none of the DI parents had told their child. A year later,
interestingly, a comparison of single and married recipients of DI did not
show significant differences in attitudes towards disclosure at the time of
recruitment, but more single women said that they intended to tell the
child of the means of their conception. A New Zealand study (Daniels
and Taylor, 1993) showed that 30 per cent of 181 respondents gave their
children information about their conception. Of the parents who had not
told them yet, 77 per cent intended to tell their child later.

As for the children's view, there are few systematic studies of DI or
oocyte donation and children's attitudes to anonymity or disclosure of
the donor's identity, although we are all aware of specific cases where the
frustration of not being able to know the donor's identity has led to a
strong feeling of deprivation in the offspring.

Analogies have been made with adopted children and, in France, with
the fate of children born 'under X', which means that even the mother's
name is not available to the child. Whether this situation in which
children are abandoned before being adopted is indeed similar, especially psychologically, to that of children desired and sought for by
extraordinary means, even before their conception through gamete donation, is still a matter for debate; one's inclination is to think that the two
situations are very different, at least psychologically. As for adopted children, recent research shows sex differences between searchers and
non-searchers in a fascinating study, which could be used as a model

when children of AHR techniques ask for information from the HFEA in the future, even though the situation is different (Howe and Feast, 2000).

The donors themselves also have a voice to be heard, because the birth of a child would not be possible without their generosity. A study of oocyte donors in Finland showed that 59 per cent thought that children ought to be told of their origin whereas a third thought that they should be given identifying information (Soderstrom-Antilla et al., 2001).

Another important matter is what specific information will be available in the future for informed offspring. In the UK, some of the information from the registration forms of donors will probably be imparted. The form contains a pen portrait from the donors, although this is not compulsory. The following results come from a study (Shenfield et al., 1998) at the Lister IVF unit: a total of 585 women donated oocytes between August 1991 and end of June 1997 in London. Of those, 389 women donated anonymously and 196 were known donors (66.6 vs 33.3 per cent). Only 1.1 per cent of known donors responded to the request for a pen portrait, an expectable result if anonymity is not part of the donation/recipient equation. This was significantly lower than the response from anonymous donors, where 8.9 per cent responded to this question. The response to other questions (profession, interests) may also be given to the child in the future, and these have to be completed by the donor.

Here again, there is certainly no consensus at the European level. In France, where legislation is due to be revised, the emphasis has been on modifications of the constraints on embryo research, and the matter of gamete anonymity has barely been raised. In the UK, lawyers are readying themselves to prepare challenges to anonymity under the Human Rights legislation implemented in October 2000. Whether this would push determined parents to maintain secrecy in an even higher proportion than is already the case is impossible to fathom. Therefore, major questions to decide where future legal changes are contemplated are, first, the amount and details of anonymous information to be given to the offspring and, second, whether anonymity should eventually be dispensed with. Meanwhile, the UK should at least ready itself for 2008, because, according to the HFE Act 1990, any child who thinks that he or she may be the product of assisted reproduction (licensed) treatment may, at 18, or younger if about to marry, find out from the HFEA whether he or she is not about to marry a half-sibling, or request the anonymous information per the directions yet to be implemented.

The Australian state of Victoria has set up a gamete donor register (ITA website, 2001, www.ita.org.au). The register is voluntary and will include information on donors of genetic material, and the resulting children. The register is thought to be the first of its kind in the world, and will allow the offspring of donated sperm, eggs or embryos to contact their donors. For the first time, children under the age of 18 will be able to get in touch with their donor 'parent'. But the voluntary register will take applications only from children born from donated gametes or embryos since 1988. The Victoria Infertility Treatment Authority (ITA) will oversee a programme in which donors would be able to apply to have different levels of information about them made available to donor offspring. The chief executive of the ITA said that, 'they can apply to put in a name, . . . to say they want to meet their genetic counterpart, they can send in a photo'. Supporters of the new register say that they will campaign to have similar registers in all states and territories of Australia. But some groups have said that most parents who conceive using donated gametes would not be interested in applying to join the register. A specialist of the Queensland Fertility Group said that many parents do not tell their children how they were conceived, others do not want contact with the donor and a voluntary register would probably do little to change this.

One's interpretation of Article 8, with the respect to the privacy of all parties involved, is reassured by the word 'voluntary'. Indeed all this may push prospective parents to cross state boundaries, although, on the contrary, this may prompt them to be open and dispense with the usual secrecy, on the grounds that they would rather the child learnt the facts from them than from an anonymous official body, even if counselling is provided. To return to what the offspring will be told, the final and most complex question is whether anonymous information is going to be, on the whole, gratifying or more frustrating than no information. It must be suspected that the answer will not be monolithic, but at last we may have some evidence resulting from this social experiment. Arguably, what may matter most to the child to be is the concern of the future parents of the prospective child, i.e. the recipient couple, because their attitude will directly influence the well-being and welfare of the child. The fact that we still have no evidence that the outcome is not generally at least as good as that of naturally conceived offspring is reassuring, but we must not forget our (ethical) responsibility to these children as a profession, and indeed our (legal) duty of care whether general or specific as it is in UK law.

It is indeed our duty to look prospectively and reflect on different approaches. For the time being, it seems that democratic openness to different approaches in families and the respect of their privacy favours a two-strand approach (Pennings, 1997), with all the consequences for the children for whom we are jointly responsible.

Sex selection

Sex selection for medical reasons is not discussed here, because for the time being it may be the only way to avoid having a child who would suffer from a serious disease such as haemophilia. Sex selection for social reasons is, however, in the opinion of this author, an issue of discrimination. The Nobel prize-winning economist has estimated that a hundred million women are 'missing' (Sen, 1990). This results less from foetal prenatal sex screening by ultrasonography than from infanticide (by exposure or drowning), child abuse (by food deprivation or unequal distribution of food and education between the sexes) and murder (brides burning for insufficient dowries). Child abuse of any kind is not confined to societies where it is culturally unfortunate to be a female, but sex selection by prenatal means is condoned by some on the grounds that it may prevent many such criminal acts (a consequentialist argument).

Before discussing preimplantation means, it must be stressed that, if prenatal sex determination is performed with a view to terminate a pregnancy of the wrong sex, this is actually in most legislations an illegal abortion. The Canadian example shows, however, how some women cross the border to the USA to have foetal sex determination and return for a termination of pregnancy in Canada if the child is of the unwanted sex (Nisker and Jones, 1997). Furthermore, when preimplantation sex diagnosis is allowed, a Code of Practice will generally ensure that it is performed for a medical reason and not for a social one. Let us therefore discuss here only preconceptual means of sex selection.

One may use several ethical theories in order to analyse this dilemma. First, the utilitarian argument: it may be forceful if one could prove that the moral cost–benefit analysis to society is actually in favour of this pragmatic solution in order to prevent more serious harm, but the cost to society is of reinforcing discriminatory attitudes.

As stated by the anthropologist Strathern, 'it is worth asking whether making it acceptable to select one sex in preference to another at the moment of conception will make it easier or harder to promote anti-discriminatory measures in other areas of life' (M. Strathern, oral communication at BMA meeting in 1993).

The duty-based argument (deontology) states that the Kantian principle of universality of any 'reasonable' moral rule means that we cannot accept sex selection as a luxurious item 'of fancy' in affluent societies and as an economic necessity of less affluent countries (Egozcue, 1993). Whatever the reasons for following a moral rule, they should be the same in any culture or environment. Indeed, the medical profession has always prided itself that it would treat equally and without discrimination anyone in need, regardless of creed or background.

Finally, the rights-based argument is perhaps the strongest argument against sex selection, the most modern one and a political rather than a philosophical one. We are considering here a fundamental issue of human rights based on the non-discrimination on grounds of sex, religion or phenotype enshrined in both the Universal Declaration of Human Rights of 1948, and the European Convention of Human Rights of 1950. These human rights are paramount and 'trump' any other claimed right (Dworkin, 1991). They may also be enshrined in national legislation.

One may also raise the question of whether a compromise is possible. Pennings (1996) has proposed the notion of family balancing: this means offering the technique only in favour of the outnumbered sex, and not if the family is balanced and not for the first child; but this still leaves us with the question 'is sex selection inherently sexist?'. It is of note that the issue of sex selection in Turkey has led to intense debate, with the conclusion that 'gender should never be treated as a disorder' (Kalaca and Akin, 1997) – a conclusion already reached elsewhere (Shenfield, 1994) – 'gender (is not) a serious handicap worthy of termination' or selection.

Let us think about the children, and whether it would be a benefit to be born in such a society where prejudice has become the norm, and hope (against hope?) that any child may be born in a tolerant society, accepting of all the differences of phenotype, sex and disabilities, and keen to protect human rights for all. Indeed, the author would interpret human rights as the modern version of the Kantian imperative, whether in its first or second formulation (i.e. universality of all moral rules, and treating any person as an end in him- or herself and not as a means).

Do all cases of sex selection send the message that life of a certain sex is more valuable than life of another? Internationally, children of the male sex are preferred (Kumar, 1996; Kalaca and Akin, 1997). Even in cases where sex selection is used for 'family completion' or 'family balance', there is a marked trend for families to select a male child as firstborn, which arguably has negative consequences for females and society as a whole. Do all sex-selection techniques perpetuate the existence of women as second-class citizens (Shenfield, 1994)?

In a 1991 survey of health professionals encountering abortion, Evans and colleagues concluded: 'Abortion for sex selection violates equality in a radical way. Also, sex is not a disease, and to abort for sex is a precedent to eugenics.' These American authors feel limits should be placed on those 'assisting with abortions or selective terminations' (Evans et al., 1991). Although Western cultures remain patriarchal, most condemn as misogyny such deliberate femicidal practices as sex selection abortion. Regardless of the personal or cultural motivation, the message sex selection for non-medical reasons sends to the broader society is the suboptimal worth of women and abrogation of responsibility to preserve human life.

Conclusion

The discussion of these few dilemmas has implications at national and international levels, as do many others in our specialty. However, the individual dimension is often the most poignant, and this is the one that practitioners certainly face in their daily practice. Nevertheless, international comparisons with the study of different sociocultural approaches help us to challenge dogma, a very sane attitude when one keeps in mind Wittgenstein's definition of philosophy, applicable to ethics: 'philosophy is not a doctrine, but an activity with the aim to logically clarify one's thinking'. The interdisciplinary approach also allows us to take into account the welfare of the future child, with the invaluable help of psychologists and counsellors, especially those who specialise in family dynamics.

Finally, a word about the law: according to Bernard Dickens (1997), 'law and ethics interact as normative systems which may overlap or conflict . . . . Ethics frames the law within which law is voluntarily obeyed'. Added to this is the weight of culture and tradition, as seen in India where the law against social sex selection has failed in practice, and the opposite example of Sweden where couples who do not wish to use a known donor seek treatment outside the country. This is a final plea for debate and information before any modifications that may happen in the UK, with the current consultation document on gamete donation and knowledge of genetic identity for resulting children.

References

Broderick P, Walker I (1995) Information access and donated gametes: how much do we know about who wants to know? Human Reproduction 10: 3338.

Cook R, Golombok S, Bish A et al. (1995) Disclosure of donor insemination: parental attitudes. American Journal of Orthopsychiatry 65: 549–559.

Daniels KR, Taylor K (1993) Secrecy and openness in donor insemination. Politics Life Sciences, 12: 200–203.

Dickens B (1997) Interfaces of assisted reproduction, ethics and law. In: Shenfield F, Sureau C (eds), Ethical Dilemmas in Assisted Reproduction. New York: Parthenon.

Dworkin G (1991) Taking Rights Seriously. London: Duckworth.

Egozcue J (1993) Sex selection: why not? Human Reproduction 8: 1777.

Evans M, Drugan A, Bottoms SF et al. (1991) Attitudes on the ethics of abortion, sex selection and selective pregnancy termination amongst health care professionals, ethicists, and clergy likely to encounter such situations. American Journal of Obstetrics and Gynecology 164: 1092–1099.

Golombok S, Breaways A, Cook R et al. (1996) The European study of assisted reproduction families: family functioning and child development. Human Reproduction 11: 2324–2331.

Gollancz D (2001) Donor insemination: a question of rights. Human Fertility 4: 164–167.

Gottlieb C, Lalos O, Lindblad F (2000) Disclosure of donor insemination to the child: the impact of Swedish legislation on couple's attitudes. Human Reproduction 15: 2052–2056.

Howe D, Feast J (2000) Adoption, Search and Reunion. London: The Children's Society Publishing Department.

Human Fertilisation and Embryology Authority (1994) Third Annual Report. London: HFEA.

Human Fertilisation and Embryology Authority (2001) Fifth Code of Practice. London: HFEA.

IFFS (2001) IFFS surveillance 01. Fertility and Sterility 76 (suppl 2): 178.

Kalaca C, Akin A (1997) Sex selection debate. Human Reproduction 10: 1631–1632.

Kumar TCA (1996) Legislation on reproductive technology in India. Human Reproduction 11: 685.

Nisker J, Jones M (1997) The ethics of sex selection. In: Shenfield F, Sureau C (eds), Ethical Dilemmas in Assisted Reproduction. New York: Parthenon.

Pennings G (1996) Ethics of sex selection for family balancing: family balancing as a morally acceptable application of sex selection. Human Reproduction 11: 2339–2343.

Pennings G (1997) The double track policy for donor anonymity. Human Reproduction 12: 2839–2844.

Pennings G, Liebaers I (2002) Creating a child to save another. HLA matching of siblings by means of PGD. In Shenfield F, Sureau C (eds), Ethical Dilemmas in Assisted Reproduction. New York: Parthenon.

Polkinghorne Report (1989) Review on the guidance on the research use of foetuses and foetal material. Cmnd 762. London: HMSO.

Rodriguez del Pozo P (1994) Paying donors and the ethics of blood supply. Journal of Medical Ethics 20: 31–35.

Schover LR, Rothmann SA, Collins RL (1992) The personality and motivation of semen donors: a comparison with oocyte donors. Human Reproduction 7: 575–579.

Sen A (1990) More than 100 million women are missing. New York Review of Books 20/12/1990.

Seve L (1994) Pour une critique de la raison bioethique. In: Respect. Paris: editions Odile Jacob, pp. 144–146.

Shenfield F (1994) Sex selection, why not? Human Reproduction 9: 569.

Shenfield F (2002) Cloning: therapeutic, reproductive or not at all? In: Shenfield F, Sureau C (eds), Ethical Dilemmas in Assisted Reproduction. New York: Parthenon.

Shenfield F, Steele SJ (1997) What are the effects of anonymity and secrecy on the welfare of the child in gamete donation? Human Reproduction 12: 392–5.

Shenfield F, Abdalla HI, Latarche E (1998) What shall we tell the children of oocyte donation? Human Reproduction 13: 1106–1109.

Soderstrom-Antilla V, Foudila T, Ripatti UR, Siegberg R (2001) Embryo donation: outcome and attitudes among embryo donors and recipients. Human Reproduction 16: 1120–1128.

Titmuss R (1971) The GIFT Relationship: From human blood to social policy. London: Allen & Unwin.

Weil E (1992) Le secret pour qui? Contraception Fertilité Sexologie 20: 737–740.

CHAPTER 3

Ethical issues – the major faiths: a personal view

JIM RICHARDS

The deep longing many couples have for children provides a drive which, when it leads to the birth of a child, gives rise to understandable pride and outpourings of love. This creation by parents, which brings with it the satisfaction of natural selfish ends, is also hugely important for society at large. Put simply, without that drive we would not survive. This is one reason why society is concerned about the creation of new life. It is, however, also concerned about the establishment of families and secular society has rules, which may well vary from country to country, about the circumstances and conditions by which people form the next generation. As the family is seen as the key building block of civic society, which helps determine the shape of a particular society, there is a legitimate societal interest, not just in whether there are sufficient numbers of children, but also about the key unit, the family, in which they are cared for and loved.

Behind these secular rules, where matters of age, consanguinity and other factors are legislated for, there will be an ethical system. Dependent on the particular culture or cultures of a country, these will to a greater or lesser extent be influenced by religious beliefs, acting in both a historical and a contemporary context. Moreover, sometimes these beliefs may be in conflict with those of the particular state where the belief, and increasingly beliefs, are held and those holding these beliefs will, to varying degrees, both influence and be influenced by the secular rules of the state. Indeed, for many believers, it will be seen as their duty to do as much as possible to convince their host state of the rightness of their position and thereby influence legislation.

Such a stance is taken because the belief systems and ethical views held by those with a faith do not, in their view, spring from the state but come from a divine being and the divinely inspired writings of that particular faith. It is to these that believers will turn to seek answers to ethical problems. The aim of this chapter, therefore, is to consider the different forms of assisted human reproduction and to consider how some religious communities, and within the Christian faith also how certain denominations, have wrestled with the ethical dilemmas created by the new reproductive technologies. Space does not permit a comprehensive examination of all the faiths/religions, or indeed their many offshoots, but it is hoped that the variety of beliefs and their resulting ethical positions will be sufficient to serve as examples of the commonalities as well as key differences of approach. The aim is also to suggest to believers and non-believers alike that the examination of the views of these faiths can assist in the development of their own positions in this area.

The ethical issues surrounding assisted human reproduction are ever present. Religious communities are grappling with them all the time and their guidance is available not just to believers but also to the wider society. The strength of these views stems in large part from how the religious communities look to their founding beliefs and principles for guidance in the light of today's knowledge. The pain of infertility on an individual level will also be considered, alongside the wider needs of society.

The major religious groups readily concur with the Islamic belief that children are a blessing that it is in Allah's gift to grant or deny and, if the latter is ordained, the community should be there to be concerned and to comfort. Such a stance of considering the needs of all of society in the light of a divinely inspired belief system runs counter to the growth of Western individualism and moral relativism. This is discussed later, but the issues involved are very real and the following examples indicate the need for both debate and guidance.

One aspect of the donation of sperm that is not often discussed is the number of times a male is able to donate his sperm, and therefore potentially how many children he may 'father'. This was highlighted recently in a report of a donor who is thought to be a carrier of Opitz's syndrome (Rogers, 2001). This rare condition often leads to prolonged illness and early death. The donor had fathered 43 children via a London clinic, doing so before the 1990 Human Fertilisation and Embryology Act restricted the maximum number of children that may be fathered by any one donor to 10 – a figure that some might still consider to be unusually high, given the size of families today. The clinic does not intend to contact this donor or the parents of the other children. The issues here include the giving of sperm for financial gain, fathers whose children cannot be contacted when adult, the weakening of the unifying and procreative aspects of marriage, and the secrecy and therefore high possibility of deception in such processes.

A further news item highlights the growth, prevalence and acceptability of surrogacy in California (O'Driscoll, 2001). In it, the surrogates are portrayed as 'just normal mums who really enjoy being pregnant' and they explain to their children that they are 'lending their womb for another person'. Surrogacy is discussed more fully below, but the main issues to emerge are the implications for life-long commitment of responsible maternal love, fidelity in marriage, and the rights of the child born, as well as the surrogate's existing children, who see their brother or sister taken away by another 'mummy and daddy'. The transaction is also commercial and almost invariably of rich people hiring a relatively poorer person's womb.

Different ethical issues arise when parents seek to create a child instrumentally, not so much because they desire that child for his or her own sake, but because this additional child may enable an existing sibling to survive. One such case, of a British couple who received treatment in the USA, involved the recovery from leukaemia of their 4-year-old, who had a 25 per cent possibility of relapse (Meek, 2001). The conventional way of treating such a condition is to seek a compatible bone marrow donor. This search can be fruitless, even within the family. However, IVF techniques now enable embryos to be screened before implantation so that the desired match can be made. Stem cells from the umbilical cord are removed at birth, frozen and then donated to the sibling, should the need arise. Opposition to this procedure is based on the judgement that, by screening and then discarding embryos, the prime concern is the compatibility of a particular embryo for the existing child not the embryos themselves. In other words, a child is created (and others destroyed) not for his or her own sake but for the potential usefulness to a sibling. In the particular case, 22 embryos were created over two cycles, the second cycle leading to a pregnancy. As with surrogacy, this is a course of action available only for the relatively wealthy, at a reputed cost of £30 000.

Marriage and the creation of children

Within Christianity, when a man and woman marry (each created as they are in the image of God) they 'become partners in a divine undertaking' (Encyclical Letter, 1995). It is also a covenant relationship, where a couple make a promise at the point of becoming one, to stay together till death. Moreover, the grace of matrimony is not just there on the wedding day; it is something that continues throughout married life, providing a basis for the building of the couple's love for each other, for God and for children born to them. As in marriage both husband and wife give to each other unconditional love in total trust, marriage is largely seen as indissoluble. As a model of how to relate one to another, marriage is, as Cardinal Hume wrote in 1984, not 'just about believers, it is about people generally. The Christian view of marriage as a life-long commitment of love between husband and wife in fact articulates the deepest, more genuine instincts of people in love'. In Western society, where an increasingly high value is placed on personal freedom, Christian marriage should not be seen as an infringement of freedom; rather it is based on constancy and commitment, one for the other. Marriage is seen as 'An experience of surrender without absorption, or service without compulsion' (Coffey, 2000).

Unsurprisingly this view of marriage is shared by the Jewish faith as both derive much of their teaching from the Old Testament and both believe that we are both body and soul. There is also a Jewish concept of an intimate personal partnership of the husband and wife with God in creating new life (Jakobovits, 1975). The book of *Genesis* states that it was God's will that man and woman be united, and this is reinforced by the prophet Malachi reminding married people of their promise to be faithful to each other.

There has, for many years, been a mutual interchange of ideas, within the Western moral tradition, among Christianity, Islam and Judaism (see also Schenker, 2000). As Brendan Soane (1988) observed 'Even Chaucer's Doctor of Phisik had the great Arabs on his bookshelf'. Therefore it is not surprising that in Islam, as with Christianity, marriage is the context in which children should be reared but, rather than having the Judaeo-Christian basis of a unitive covenanting relationship with God, it is seen more as a legally binding agreement and mutual commitment to lead a life in accordance with the faith. The lifelong exclusivity of the Judaeo-Christian tradition has its exceptions in Islam, given the possibilities, albeit limited, of polygamy. Broadly, there are two situations where this may happen: a woman, who becomes a widow, perhaps at time of war, may be married as a type of act of charity. In a similar vein, a divorced woman with children may also be married and she and her family given shelter. Polygamy is also a possibility where a wife may not be able to meet sexual, or other needs, of her husband.

In Buddhism, as with Islam, marriage is not a blessed state but there is a belief in mutual faithfulness. This stems from a key ethical precept of the avoidance of misconduct, with unfaithfulness being, by definition, misconduct. One should also not cause harm by one's actions. This underlies the need for commitment to one's spouse and also the need to care for children of the marriage, who may be hurt by adultery or separation.

How a child is physically created is also of key importance. There is broad agreement in all faiths with the view that a child has the right to be carried in his or her mother's womb and brought up within marriage. In the security and love of the parents, children develop their own identity and reach maturity. However, how this is interpreted, where variance is allowed and, crucially, when human life begins forms much of what follows.

The status of the human embryo

In 1996 the General Assembly of the Church of Scotland debated a wide-ranging report (Easton, 1996) on IVF and embryology and passed several 'deliverances' based on its comprehensive and thoughtful contents. Of particular relevance were those that affirmed 'the sanctity of the embryo from conception', that 'its special nature be recognised in law' and that 'given the law already stated that research on embryos be allowed up to 14 days, any extension was to be opposed' and that the Assembly recognized the different views held on the 'ethical acceptability of IVF and embryo research'.

The above echoed the recommendations of and discussions within the report. Most noteworthy in this regard is where the report examined what they described as a 'Conflict of Obligation'. This led them to state that: 'a certain latitude of judgement is to be expected among Christians'. Strong convictions lie behind the different positions adopted. In these circumstances, it believes that it is not right to make dogmatic pronouncements, or to burden further the consciences 'of those working in the field or of Christians who believe it right to receive certain treatments for infertility'.

This Anglican view is echoed by Baptists in the UK, where there is no hierarchy and where it is rare for the Baptist Union to make policy statements. On this subject, however, it has produced material for making a judgement (Coffey, 2000). In it, it recognises that there is a broad range of opinion about when human life begins and what protection it should be afforded during its various stages. Furthermore, although the embryo is to be protected 'the extent of such protection is debated'.

Similarly, within the Jewish tradition, the embryo is accorded some degree of protection and its potential for life is not to be extinguished except in the most exceptional of circumstances, related to what have been described as 'the most substantial of medical conditions' involving risks to the mother's health. Broadly speaking the longer the unborn child is *in utero*, the greater the protection afforded to that child. The unborn child therefore 'enjoys a very sacred title to life' but it does not have full human inviolability (Dunstan and Seller, 1988).

Islam also recognises the special nature of the potential human person from the point of conception and it is only in extreme situations, in the same way as described immediately above, that termination of that potential should occur. Termination of life in the womb also assumes greater seriousness as the pregnancy proceeds as 'it is then ready to receive life. Disturbing it is a crime. When it develops further . . . abortion is a greater crime. When it acquires a soul and its creation is complete, the crime becomes even more serious' (Hewitt, 1998).

There is a similar recognition of the importance of life created at the time of conception in Buddhism: 'When that junction of the father's sperm, the mother's ovum, and the consciousness to be reborn takes place, there arises, in dependence on the volitional activities, sentience, the first tiny flash of consciousness in the single cell of the embryo' (Subhuti, 1985). Life created is also to be seen as precious, and harming or destroying life, at whatever its stage of development, is to be avoided.

We thus have in the above a belief in the special status of the embryo, namely that this form of life is protected but not to the degree of total inviolability. However, the Roman Catholic Church bestows such a status on life from the point of conception. Its position is stated unequivocally: 'The human being is to be respected and treated as a person from the moment of conception' and therefore has 'the inviolable right of every innocent human being to life' as 'it would never be made human if it were not human already' (Encyclical Letter, 1995). This new life, although created by man and woman, is separate from each and will develop in its own unique way. Cardinal Cormac Murphy-O'Connor (2001) explained this by drawing an analogy between an embryo and an adult in a coma, the period of 'coma' ending at a usually predetermined time. Just as a person in a coma can be helped or harmed and certainly has interests, so too does the unborn child.

The natural occurrence of twinning, which occurs when the fertilized egg divides at about 14 days after conception, is used as a reason to deny the embryo special protection or a moral status. The argument runs that there is this time-limited potential to split into two individuals. Therefore, until it is clear that there is going to be one or two embryos, it cannot be said that an individual exists because how can one person become two?

This position is countered by the observation that far less than one per cent of naturally conceived embryos become twins. It should also be realised that an embryo is programmed from the start to separate and become twins. The logic of the position, where an embryo is not afforded protection until the possibility of twinning has passed, is that it is treated as if there is no person present. Similarly it is argued that, as a large number of fertilized embryos are naturally aborted, they do not therefore have a right to protection at that early stage. But the counter-argument points out that when many people die in natural disasters their loss is mourned, not just by those who knew them, but often by many others far away. The deceased will be seen as having value in their own right as human beings. Likewise, just because an embryo is naturally aborted does not mean that it is not of intrinsic value and can be destroyed.

Finally, there is what might be referred to as the developmental or continuity argument. From the point of conception, the embryo is in a continuous state of growth and change. In its early stages, it is merely a group of undifferentiated cells and quite unlike a human form. It is only later in the unborn child's life that this child can be said to have achieved personhood.

The difficulties of this position are that it is impossible in any scientific way to point to a particular stage when the status of personhood occurs. It can be decided only arbitrarily. Moreover, such a view reduces human personhood to what someone can do or what they are capable of doing. It also ignores the point that the totality of the unborn child's genetic code is within the embryo, and that its development started *in utero* and continues after birth (Murphy-O'Connor, 2001).

The major religions are in broad agreement that it is ethically in order to carry out therapeutic procedures on the human embryo while *in utero*. They do, however, make certain provisos, the key element being that the procedures should be directed towards healing and the survival of the embryo. Furthermore, such treatments should not be applied unless with the full and informed consent of the parents.

In the Christian tradition there are two theological issues at play. Healing is seen 'as part of God's gracious provision' (Congregation for the Doctrine of the Faith, 1987). By God's providence we may be healthy and be healed to help us grow in faith. That is why, for the Christian doctor, it is not just about relieving suffering and trying to make someone well, but about the person being treated as someone made in the image of God and helping to preserve the divine gift of life.

In a similar vein, Islam preaches the good that comes from treating disease and illness and this in turn is linked to its encouragement of scientific progress. Such progress, if successful and carried out within the regulations, will have the effect of warding off harm, this being one of the main aims of Islamic Shari'ah. But as with Christianity there is providence, summed up in the sentence, 'Anything He does is for a purpose that He alone knows' (Islam Online, 2001).

Warnock and moral relativism

It will be clear that the status given by a belief system to the unborn child will play a large part in determining views about particular forms of assisted human reproduction. First, however, it will be helpful to examine briefly one further area – certain ethical criticisms of the influential Warnock Report (1984).

The key secular report on assisted human reproduction is the 1984 Warnock Report. It has framed much of the debate in the UK and was a major influence on subsequent legislation, most notably the Human Fertilisation and Embryology Act 1990 and the establishment of the

Human Fertilisation and Embryology Authority (HFEA). The Report has, however, been heavily criticized, not least for its avoidance of certain ethical issues (Atkinson, 1994). Thus, Warnock failed to answer the key question about when a person is created: 'Instead of trying to answer the question directly we have therefore gone straight to the question of how it is right to treat the human embryo'. Such an approach left the field open for research and experimentation on embryos with a majority of the Committee voting for this on both 'spare' embryos and those created just for experimentation up to 14 days from conception. Some argued strongly against this with, for instance, Sir John Peel (1987), a former President of the Royal College of Gynaecologists stating that this arbitrary cut-off 'has no real scientific, moral or practical basis'. He also pointed out that 'None of the distinguished moral philosophers or Churchmen who had publicly taken up conservative positions on the ethical issues under discussion was invited to serve on Warnock' (Warnock, 1987) – a position that exists today in Warnock's offspring, the HFEA (Ahmed, 2001). The results can be seen in the HFEA's stance on the controversial practice of what are commonly known as 'baby gender' clinics, which enable parents to predetermine the sex of their child via laboratory methods. The HFEA reportedly stated: 'We need to know whether public opinion has moved on and certainly where the science has moved to'. Also implicit in the Report was the view that conception should no longer be seen as a gift, but that parenthood is now to be regarded as a right, rather than a vocation.

From this standpoint the notion of the embryo develops as a technically contrived product, often one for which we pay, not one conceived spontaneously – hence the ease with which we discard spare embryos, experiment with them, store them and even neglect to reply, with regard to the last, when asked by a clinic what the 'owners' of the frozen embryos want done with them (discarded, used by the parents, used by other potential parents or for experimentation). Moreover, rather than calling up a body of ethical opinion by which to judge a particular act, Warnock went down the road of either advocating the stance that private personal preference was allowable, or that the will of the majority be exercised through Parliament. Warnock was 'reluctant to appear to dictate on matters of morals' and adopted 'a steady and general point of view' – this latter phrase being almost totally meaningless.

Those who advocate assisted human reproduction, which as a consequence may result in the destruction of human embryos, or the introduction of third parties into a marriage through gamete donation, argue not only that the end justifies the means, but also that most of the population favour these procedures. Warnock maintained that it was possible to be 'a living human being' without the status of personhood.

Warnock, therefore, saw personhood as something that could be socially defined. The difficulty here is that social definitions, enacted through Parliament, or brought about by the practice of institutions or individuals, can lead to a lack of protection of the most vulnerable in society. In the present instance that is the embryo, but in other circumstances it might be elderly or infirm people or those with severe handicaps, whose 'quality of life' is judged to be so poor that it should end. Perhaps it was with this in mind that a minority view on Warnock held that: 'It is in our view wrong to create something with the potential for becoming a human person and then deliberately to destroy it.' Thus, if we regard all human life as having a moral claim on us, at whatever its stage of development, every human is our neighbour with a claim on our love. That sort of thinking was absent from the majority view in Warnock.

The majority view on the Warnock report was arrived at on the basis of moral relativism. This position places a high value on personal freedom, and thereby ignores universal truths, with morality becoming subjective and changeable. In this way society rejects a moral system based on commonly held values, and moral positions are formed on the basis of an individual's views in relation to his or her own situation. However, this placing of personal autonomy at the pinnacle of values can lead us to reject each other. We have arrived at the position of making it legal to destroy embryos because we have argued as a society that the life of an unborn child is only a relative good to be compared with other goods. For instance, by experimenting on embryos we may find the cause of disease in others, or by creating a surplus of embryos we can implant the fittest and destroy the remainder. This was essentially the view of Warnock, which led to the legislation providing a permissive framework within which it is possible to make an individualized decision. Moreover, because this position has been legislated for via Parliament, it also expresses the will of the majority. A moral relativist stance argues that the State, through its laws, should not create a situation where the morality espoused within the legislation is higher than that with which most of the citizens would agree. The relativist would also point out that, if a law is passed that does not have majority backing, it will fall into disrepute and people will either directly disobey it or, in relation to assisted human reproduction, go to countries that allow procedures banned here.

Thus, on the basis of freedom of choice, people should be able to devise their own morality, and it is not the role of the State to impose an ethical position on its citizens. Further, where legislation has to be passed, it should be in such a way that it allows as much freedom as possible for the individual, so long as it does not impinge on the freedom of others. Therefore, the parameters of possible ethical positions are bound by law rather than by an overriding morality. In this way we are able to coexist peacefully and tolerantly in a pluralistic democratic society. The alternative, based on an overriding moral structure from which laws should be derived, is seen as leading to the creation of an authoritarian and intolerant society.

Of course, what we have created is the intolerance of the majority, which, acting through democratic structures, allows the position that permits the killing of unborn human life. Democracy is not moral in itself. It is a means by which desired ends may be achieved. It is therefore moral in so far as the means and ends are moral. From a broadly Christian perspective, a democracy has to be underpinned by enduring values, which cannot be overturned by a majority. One such value should be something that makes clear that it is always wrong and should never be allowed in law to kill an innocent human being at whatever stage of that person's life. When the most vulnerable can in law be dispensed with, we have a position in which the wishes of the powerful are those that hold sway. In such circumstances, this is a subversion of democracy. The principal duty of Government is not to ensure that individuals be allowed as much freedom as possible, but 'to safeguard the enviable rights of the human person, and to facilitate the performance of his duties' (Encyclical Letter, 1963). To be safeguarded in this way means that all humans are treated as equal in this respect. The State should create laws and structures where all can be protected on the basis of our common equality. Arguably, it is a negation of the democratic ideal for a State not to safeguard equally all those within it.

Particular forms of assisted human reproduction

Artificial insemination by husband

In circumstances where it is not possible for husband and wife to conceive naturally, this difficulty may be overcome by artificial insemination by husband (AIH), whereby sperm is externally collected and then artificially inserted into the wife. Within Islam such a procedure is not objected to because it involves just the husband and wife, albeit with medical help, and therefore the lineage of the child is clear. It may be argued that such procedures are an interference with Allah's plan but this is countered by infertility being seen as a 'disease' or 'defect' and our responsibility to try to overcome it.

A similar position, with regard to AIH, is held by Jewish law, and by many Christians. The former stresses the care needed in the procedures so that the biological mother and father can be identified with absolute certainty. Among the latter, many believe that AIH does not breach the sanctity of marriage, that the child produced is derived from the love the couple have for each other and that it does not preclude sexual intimacy.

However, the Catholic Church takes a different view, based on their teachings on marriage and sexual intercourse within it. The two are the 'inseparable connection, willed by God and unable to be broken by man on his own initiative, between the two meanings of the conjugal act: the unitive meaning and the procreative meaning' (Encyclical Letter, 1963). The basis for this view comes from the belief in the unity of the human being of both body and soul. The marriage of two people is consummated through and in the bodies of husband and wife. It is in this way that they are able to become a mother and father, with their children being created as a result of the full expression of their married love.

Third-party reproduction

Donor insemination (DI) is not accepted by the major religions. Although it is recognized that it does not constitute true sexual adultery, the child is nevertheless conceived outside the marriage. It also disrupts the family relationship and, given donor anonymity, the child would be denied the right to know his or her biological father and other blood relatives. There is also the argument that, by using DI, the couple are not accepting each other as they are – 'for better or for worse'. It may also weaken their marriage bond and there is the potential for psychological harm to the child and, if the child is not told how he or she was conceived, of secrecy and lying. The last two are not a sound basis for a faith-based life. There is concern not just about the damage to relationships within the family as a result of DI, but also about adverse social repercussions.

Given the above view on DI, it can readily be understood that similar views are held when *in vitro* fertilization (IVF) is used with either donated sperm or egg. However, where the gametes are of husband and wife, the views are more varied, and debate centres on the creation of 'spare' embryos and foetal reduction. For those who agree to the possibility of this procedure, there is the view that the embryo has a moral status and should be protected, but that such protection is not absolute. They believe that there may be a higher moral demand to help infertile couples. Thus, excess embryos created *in vitro* will be allowed to die and, if multiple implantations successfully survive in pregnancy, then for those who believe abortion is justified, in exceptional circumstances, it is in order for selective reduction to occur. Islam has a concern about the destruction of the lives of embryos, each of which is seen as a unique human being. Such a practice is viewed as both inhumane and unethical.

In vitro fertilization

The Catholic Church recognises the suffering of infertility, but holds that the good that may come from the process is not sufficient to give a positive evaluation of IVF. The arguments already outlined about the unitive and procreative aspects of sexual intercourse in marriage apply equally in this instance, because the process is dependent on third parties outside the marriage. 'Such fertilisation entrusts the life and entity of the embryo into the power of doctors and biologists and establishes domination of technology over the origin and destiny of the human person' and would mean that the child so born was not created by husband and wife as 'co-operators with God for giving life to a new person' (Encyclical Letter, 1963).

To these arguments are added those concerning the concomitant processes of IVF, such as masturbation and abortion. Thus, although recognizing that IVF between husband and wife does not suffer from the other negative aspects of donor IVF, it is still seen as wrong, 'even when everything is done to avoid the death of the human embryo' (Encyclical Letter, 1963).

Surrogacy

Surrogacy might possibly be seen as a last resort method of reproduction, but just as DI is unanimously condemned by the major religions, so too is this procedure. Surrogacy raises particular moral issues, primarily related to the nature of motherhood and the child's rights in relation to the carrying mother. The particular forms of surrogacy considered here are where a married couple commission a woman to give birth to a child, where at least one or both of the gametes are those of the couple, or where either the egg or sperm is donated. In this procedure, fertilization takes place *in vitro* and the embryo is then implanted in the surrogate's womb. Such a procedure is recognized under UK law and enables the commissioning couple to apply to court to become the legal parents, extinguishing forever any rights of the birth mother and, if she is married, of her husband.

The objections to this process are numerous and lineage looms large in them. Within all major religions, it is argued that surrogacy severs the relationship between the mother and baby, relegating it to a commercial transaction. Moreover, the birth, *de facto*, involves a third party, the surrogate mother, who inevitably intrudes and indeed splits the unity of marriage. This is of particular concern for those religions that believe the bond of mother, father and child is divinely ordered. Furthermore, if either the egg or sperm is donated, 'parenthood' may be shared by up to four people: the surrogate mother, the donor of the egg or sperm, and the commissioning couple. Islam also argues that the mother who gives birth

to the child is the one most closely related to the child because she nour-
ished the child during pregnancy and suffered labour pains. Indeed, this
point has much force because, irrespective of the child's genetic inheritance, we now know that the environment of the womb and the birth
mother's disposition and health in pregnancy, and even such actions as
stroking the outside of her body, all have an impact on the child's future.
It is inaccurate therefore to consider the womb and pregnancy as a neutral space having no influence on the child as he or she grows within the
mother or as the child develops when born.

From these perspectives, surrogacy inverts motherhood because the
'good' surrogate is the one who willingly hands over her child. The 'bad'
surrogate is the one who decides to keep and cherish the child. One may
also speculate on the potential for harm to the child *in utero* in cases
where the host mother carries the child knowing that the intention is that
the child will never be hers.

The procedure also has great potential to create harm. Although the
agreement drawn up will state that the surrogate will not have sexual
intercourse with a third party, one can never be absolutely certain about
this, thus creating even more potential for confused parentage. Where a
close relative such as a sister is the surrogate, the birth mother, after legal
transfer of the baby, becomes the child's 'aunt'.

There have been a number of reported instances where the surrogate
has refused to hand over the baby to the commissioning parents. Under
UK law, the baby at birth belongs to the surrogate, irrespective of the
child's genetic background, the forms signed or agreements made. We
also need to consider the potential for psychological harm to any children
of the surrogate mother in seeing their mother pregnant and the baby
handed over to another. This is likely to occur whether the embryo has
resulted from the egg and sperm of the commissioning couple, or when
one or both were donated. Such scientific niceties cannot easily be
explained to a young child. The child will have seen their mother pregnant, going to hospital and then returning without a baby because the
baby has been 'given away'. A child of tender years may wonder whether
he or she will also be given away. Of course, explanations can be provided, but they are very much for the adult world and are unlikely to speak
to a child's need to know that mothers love and care for their children forever. Older children may grow up seeing motherhood as a commercial
transaction, not one based on love and life-time commitment. There is
also, as with donor *in vitro*, the issue of potential secrecy. Will the child
be told of his or her conception or birth? If not, then the legally created
family unit acts as a lie. We need also to consider the negation of the dignity of the child, which is inherent in surrogacy, where the child is an
object dependent on a commercial transaction.

Cloning

The present position in the UK is that embryonic stem cell experimentation, research and therapeutic cloning is legal. However, it is not legal to create an embryo and bring it to full term as a child. There is a growing opinion that there may well be other jurisdictions that might eventually allow the cloning of a person. Even so-called therapeutic cloning has its critics, on the basis that life has been created and, as with surplus embryos, their life is ended and, 'quite frankly, it is not therapeutic for the clone' (Murphy-O'Connor, 2001). Furthermore, if cloning leads to birth there is the inevitability of separating the creation of life from an act of love. It also creates a gross distortion in the role of parenthood, because the child created will have a relationship to those who donated to create the clone, more akin to sibling than to a parent.

Although all major religions agree that cloning to full term and birth is wrong, there is less agreement on research, experimentation and therapeutic cloning. Indeed, the levels of difference echo those within other aspects of assisted human reproduction, with the Roman Catholic Church stating that it is 'opposed in principle to any destructive interference with the early embryo' (*The Tablet*, 2002) and a Muslim view via the Islamic Medical Association holding that: 'He/she should be fully respected from the moment of conception and the fertilised egg is a sacred being.' Hindu religious leaders made similar statements to Bishop Harries' House of Lords Report on cloning. Other religious leaders put forward a gradualist view on the status of the embryo as it grows. The Bishop of Rochester for the Board for Social Responsibility of the Church of England told the Bishop Harries' Committee that his church took 'a developmental view of the emergence of personhood'. The Jewish view to the same Committee was that: 'In Jewish Law neither the foetus nor the pre-implanted embryo is a person; it is, however, human life and must be accorded the respect due to human life. Personhood, with its attendant rights and responsibilities begins at birth. Prior to birth, we have duties to both the embryo and the foetus, but these may, in certain circumstances, be overridden by other duties, namely those we owe to persons' (House of Lords, 2002).

Divine norms and pastoral needs

It would be wrong to see the upholders of the beliefs of various religions as being unfeeling or unsympathetic to the understandable desire of people to have children. It is understood that, when two people love each other, there is a natural desire to create life through that love. Not being able to conceive is therefore a great loss, but from a religious perspective the good intentions to create life by artificial means, which offend against the principles of the inalienability of all life, lead to a greater wrong. This stance forces us to address the conflict of the divine ideal and the imperfections of reality. These realities are often faced at the pastoral level, where the local religious leader comes face to face with an individual's burden or dilemma; wanting to minister to the person in their anguish, he or she has to have regard for the divine norm. These norms should not be seen as unfeeling instructions from 'head office', yet the values they espouse and the natural law that they uphold are seen as timeless.

Some religious believers will hold that the degree to which divine laws are adhered to should depend on the level of compassion and the particular situation. Others may hold that they may depend rather more on divine norm. Yet others will hold that there is a natural law and that the divine laws that stem from this cannot be disregarded, otherwise we would reach a situation where we 'allow pastoral considerations to dictate for us new sets of moral considerations' (Easton, 1996).

The concept of natural law can be explained as 'the existence of an objective moral code implanted in human nature'. Cardinal Murphy-O'Connor (2002) provided this definition when he was outlining his views on society's approaches to moral questions and the role of conscience and God's 'map'. He illuminated this concept further by using extracts from two quite different thinkers who had arrived at similar conclusions. Isaiah Berlin informs us that Albert Einstein held that here: 'Moral and aesthetic values, rules, principles cannot be derived from the sciences, which deal with what is, not with what should be; but neither are they . . . generated by differences of class, culture or race. No less than the laws of nature from which they cannot be derived, they are universal, true for men at all times, discovered by moral or aesthetic insight common to all men, and embodied in the basic principles (not the mythology) of the great world religions' (Berlin, 1975).

In the same vein, the Second Vatican Council (1979) stated: 'In the depth of his conscience man discovers a law he has not made for himself but which he must obey, a law which always call him to love and do good and shun evil, and which, when necessary, speaks clearly to his heart and says: do this; shun that. The fact is that man has within his heart a law written by God; man's dignity lies in obedience to it, and he will be judged accordingly. Conscience is the most secret core and sanctuary of man, where he finds himself alone with God, which voice can be heard in his inmost being.'

Cardinal Murphy-O'Connor (2001) pointed out, however, that the natural law should not be seen as a series of external and arbitrary prohibitions but rather as a firm foundation in our attempts to achieve

happiness and fulfilment. Given this, he suggests that our deity has provided us not with prohibitions but a 'map' and a compass in the shape of
our informed conscience. However, even though those with a faith
believe that they possess the 'real map', this does not mean that believers
have all the answers. What it does mean though is that we should not
'acquiesce in the current "post-modern" assumption that all truths are
relative and all moral precepts provisional'.

This does not detract from understanding that infertility is a great trial
and the faith community should support those so suffering. Indeed the
major faiths have an understanding of the inevitability of suffering and
loss. In the Christian tradition, this is expressed as the opportunity for
'bearing one's cross' as did Jesus and thereby having created an
opportunity for spiritual fruitfulness (Congregation for the Doctrine of
the Faith, 1987). Thus, from a seemingly negative situation there are possibilities for growth and joys to be found in other ways. Such a standpoint
may well account for the disproportionately higher number of foster car-
ers and adopters, many of whom are unable to have children of their own,
who are found in religious communities.

Conclusion

This brief and inevitably incomplete overview of the position of the major
religions in relation to assisted human reproduction cannot easily lead to
generalized conclusions, save the clear opposition to surrogacy and
human cloning. With regard to other aspects of assisted human reproduction, the differences between the official faith views are as varied as
those in wider society. However, in coming to their differing views, all the
major religions have recourse to a body of belief that guides them,
although it will have been noted that, even within one faith, for instance
Christianity, there is a wide range of views, with only the Catholic Church
affording the human being full protection from the moment of conception and fertilization – a belief that this author also holds.

Jim Richards is married with two grown-up children. He and his wife had
a third child who died in an accident as a young adult. He accepts that this
tragedy has influenced his outlook on life and the need to protect it at all
times.

References

Ahmed K (2001) Baby 'gender clinics' to face investigation. Guardian 4 November.

Atkinson D (1994) Pastoral Ethics. Oxford: Lynx Communications.

Berlin I (1995) cited in Murphy-O'Connor, Cardinal Archbishop of Westminster (2002) The real map. Briefing, Vol 32, Issue 1. Catholic Bishops' Conference of England and Wales.

Coffey D (2000) Making Moral Choices. Didcot, Oxon: The Baptist Union of Great Britain.

Congregation for the Doctrine of the Faith (1987) Instruction on Respect for Human Life with Origin. Rome: Congregation for the Doctrine of the Faith.

Dunstan GR, Seller MJ (1988) The Status of the Human Embryo. London: King Edward's Hospital Fund for London.

Easton D (1996) Pre-Conceived Ideas. A Christian Perspective of IVF and Embryology. Edinburgh: The Church of Scotland Board of Social Responsibility.

Encyclical Letter (1963) Pacem in Terris. 11 April, Rome.

Encyclical Letter (1995) Evangelium Vitae. 25 March, Rome.

Hewitt I (1998) What Does Islam Say? London: The Muslim Educational Trust.

House of Lords (2002) Select Committee Report, The status of the embryo. Hansard, as quoted in The Tablet, 9 March, pp. 31–32.

Hume, Cardinal Basil (1984) To be a Pilgrim, St Paul's. The New Testament Bible.

Islam online (2002) www.islam-online.net/completeresearch/english/Fatwa Display.asp?hFatwaID=36644.

Jakobovits I (1975) Jewish Medical Ethics. London: Bloch.

Meek J (2001) Special delivery. The Guardian 15 October.

Murphy-O'Connor C, Cardinal Archbishop of Westminster (2001) Briefing, Vol. 31, Issue 11. Bishops' Conference of England and Wales.

Murphy-O'Connor C, Cardinal Archbishop of Westminster (2002) The real map. Briefing, Vol. 32, Issue 1. Catholic Bishops' Conference of England and Wales.

O'Driscoll E (2001) What's yours is mine. The Guardian, 3 October, pp. 8–9.

Peel J (1987) Embryos and Ethics: The Warnock Report in Debate. UK: Rutherford House.

Rogers L (2001) Sperm donor children may have fatal gene. Sunday Times, 23 September.

Schenker JG (2000) Women's reproductive health: monotheistic religious perspectives. International Journal of Gynecology and Obstetrics 70(1): 77–86.

Second Vatican Council (1966) Pastoral Constitution of the Church in the Modern World. Rome: Gaudium et Spes, para 16.

Soane B (1988) Roman Catholic casuistry and the moral standing of the human embryo. In Dunstan GR, Seller MJ (eds), The Status of the Human Embryo. London: King Edward's Hospital Fund for London.

Subuthi AK (1985) The Buddhist Vision. UK: Windhorse Publications.

The Tablet (2002) House of Lords Select Committee Report. The status of the embryo. Quoted from Hansard, 9 March, pp. 31–32.

Warnock M (1984) Report of the Committee of Inquiry into Human Fertilization and Embryology, DHSS Cmnd 9314. London: HMSO.

Warnock M (1987) Embryos and Ethics: The Warnock Report in Debate. UK: Rutherford House.

CHAPTER 4

Human reproduction and human rights

DEREK MORGAN AND ROBERT G LEE

The 'reproductive revolution' raises at least two sorts of issue, on which we wish to reflect in this chapter. First, it raises a series of conceptual or theoretical questions at the interface between reproductive technology and rights, which we briefly review in the first part of the chapter. In the second part we show how assisted conception – the reproduction revolution – raises a cluster of new, practical, 'rights-based' questions of, respectively, *access* to reproductive opportunities and information attaching to these.

Reproductive rights: the stage

Many of the strongest arguments from rights-based approaches have been elegantly summarized in an accessible way by British philosopher John Harris and by American academic lawyer John Robertson.

Harris (1998), drawing explicitly and extensively on arguments developed in a more general context by the jurist Ronald Dworkin (1985, 1993, 1996, 1997), has defined and described 'a vital feature of an essentially democratic approach to reproductive choices' as lying in recognition and broad reading of the concept of 'procreative autonomy' (Harris, 1998, p. 37). As such, assisted human reproduction (AHR) can be seen as a legitimate extension of human choice, embedded in a broad sense in any genuinely democratic culture (Dworkin, 1993, pp. 166–167).

Developments in reproductive technologies have raised questions about what ought and what ought not to constrain choice in AHR. Specifically, we should ask of reproductive technologies 'is their use ethical and should access to it, or use of it, be controlled by legislation, and if so how?' (Harris, 1998, p. 34). Underlying these questions is the belief that we should not impose on those requiring medical or other assistance to conceive criteria that we do not ask, or could not be justified in asking, of those who do not need such assistance.

In this sense, arguments from reproductive rights, based on respect for procreative autonomy, demand that people should be treated in a material way as far as their procreative and parenting choices are concerned, in the same way as anyone else. Health (such as familial genetic disease), medical (such as 'primary' or 'secondary' infertility) or social reasons (same-sex choice of partner), which interfere with the ability to exercise choices that others would be able to make, should not be used as a means of discrimination between those who make one set of choices and those who make – or are forced to make – another set of choices.

Dworkin has defined the 'right of procreative autonomy' as:

> a right [of people] to control their own role in procreation unless the state has a compelling reason for denying them that control
>
> Dworkin (1993, p. 148)

and has argued that it is a protected interest under both the First and Fourteenth amendments to the US Constitution, concerning freedom of religion.

Harris takes Dworkin's expression and examination of that right in the abortion debate and asks whether it might properly be interpreted to include the right of procreative autonomy in what might be thought of as a more positive way (in assisted conception). For Harris, the right of 'procreative autonomy' would need to encompass the right:

> . . . to reproduce with the genes we chose and to which we have legitimate access, or to reproduce in ways that express our reproductive choices and our vision of the sorts of people we think it right to create.
>
> Harris (1998, p. 34)

He draws an analogy with the right of freedom of religion guaranteed in the amendments to the US Constitution. Although not spelt out in the original document, these can properly be regarded as sufficiently similar as to be relevant. *Roe v Wade* 1972 – the Supreme Court's landmark 'abortion jurisprudence' decision – itself provides an example of this. Harris suggests that the First and Fourteenth amendments are about freedoms to chose one's own way of life and to live according to one's most deeply held beliefs: '[beliefs that] are also at the heart of procreative choices' (Harris and Holm, 1998, p. 35).

In order for the argument of procreative autonomy to be trumped, it would be necessary for *any* democratic society to demonstrate that it has a *compelling* reason for denying individual citizens control over their own reproductive choices and decisions:

> In so far as the decisions to reproduce in particular ways or even using particular technologies constitute decisions concerning central issues of value . . . the state would have to show that more was at stake than the fact that a majority found the ideas disturbing or even disgusting.
>
> Harris (1998, p. 36)

These reproductive decisions are a central, almost a defining, part of moral responsibility and moral right: 'enshrining people's ability to confront the most fundamental questions about the meaning and value of their own lives for themselves, answering to their own consciences and convictions' (Dworkin, 1993, pp. 166–167).

What is required and justified is a dual caution: first in considering the acceptability of scientific 'advance' and the *use* of reproductive technologies, and second, in considering charges of unethical practices, which may in fact be baseless but which may nevertheless lead to restrictive legislation.

In contrast, Robertson (1994), drawing on reproductive debates in American constitutional law, has fashioned an account of what he has called 'procreative liberty': a version of a reproductive rights thesis grounded in procreative liberty as a negative right against state interference. This may be a right either to have children or to avoid having them. Focusing on the former 'liberty', although not applying to everything that concerns procreation, it is a primary liberty because it is central to personal identity, dignity and the meaning of one's life. A recent British case on the claim for damages for an unwanted pregnancy saw Lord Steyn advocate a position that recognises the right of parents to take decisions on family planning and, if those plans fail, their right to make their own decisions on how then to proceed:

> The law does and must respect these decisions of parents which are so closely tied to the basic freedoms and rights of personal autonomy.
>
> Steyn in *MacFarlane and another v Tayside NHS* 1999 at 976j

Lady Justice Hale, writing extra-judicially has expressed herself in similar language:

> The rights set out in Articles 8 to 12 of the European Convention on Human Rights form a coherent and related group; the right to respect for private and family life, home and correspondence; the right to freedom of

expression; the right to freedom of peaceful assembly and free association; and the right to marry and found a family. These are the very essentials of a free-thinking and free-speaking society

Hale (1997, p. 7)

Procreative liberty implies a negative right against state interference, but neither a duty to supply a service on demand, nor:

a positive right to have the state or particular persons provide the means or resources necessary to have or avoid having children.

Robertson (1994, p. 23)

Nor can there be protection against private interference, amply demonstrated by disputes over the fate of frozen embryos (see *Hecht v Superior Court of the State of California* 1993) or about abortion (*Paton v Trustees of British Pregnancy Advice Service* 1978).

Without doubt, however, social and economic circumstances have a crucial impact on the ability to access reproductive technologies and, therefore, on the exercise or enjoyment of procreative liberty. But whether the state should alleviate those conditions 'is a separate issue of social justice' (Hale, 1997). Although, as we argue below, the impact of the Human Rights Act 1998 may be likely to impose obligations that look remarkably positive.

Those who would limit reproductive choice, then, 'have the burden of showing that the reproductive actions at issue would create such substantial harm that they could justifiably be limited' (Robertson, 1994, p. 24) This distinct echo of Mill recalls Harris' claim that distaste or disgust is not in itself proper grounds for state interference with this identified claim. In Robertson's view being unmarried, homosexual, physically disabled, HIV positive or imprisoned is not sufficient grounds to override this liberty. Speculation or 'mere moral objections' cannot suffice (Robertson, 1994, p. 35). In the context of these claims, it is worth remembering that a proposal in the parliamentary debates of the Human Fertilisation and Embryology Bill 1990 to limit access to assisted conception to married couples was defeated by only one vote.

These theoretical debates highlight some of the most fertile areas for the legal manifestations of rights claims, namely various articles under the European Convention on Human Rights and its recent manifestation in British law in the Human Rights Act 1998. These may be illustrated by different types of 'access' claims under that Act, reflecting issues live and current at the time of writing. They indicate the sorts of issue that the potent mixture of human rights and human reproduction may give rise to in the forthcoming decade.

Reproductive rights: the players

Here, we consider three recent or projected cases engaging reproductive rights claims.

Sperm in the porridge: *R v Home Office ex parte (on behalf of) Mellor* 2001

Mr and Mrs Mellor, a newly wed couple, wished to start a family, but Mr Mellor is serving a life sentence in Gartree Prison. Having no right to conjugal visits, he sought assistance to enable his wife to be artificially inseminated with his sperm. Artificial insemination by husband (AIH) is not a procedure regulated by law; indeed it may require no medical intervention whatsoever. Mellor's request was thus for minimal assistance, but it was nevertheless refused. The Secretary of State stated that there was no *medical* need for artificial insemination because the request arose only from the applicant's imprisonment.

On the face of it, the rights in Article 12 to 'marry and found a family' seem absolute, whereas the right to private and family life in Article 8 is expressly subject to the restriction in Article 8(2) in the interests of:

> . . . national security, public safety, or the economic well being of the country, for the prevention of disorder or crime, for the protection of health or morals, or for the protection of the rights and freedoms of others.

The court recognised that imprisonment could entail a justifiable interference with rights under Article 8. Pointing to the limited jurisprudence of the Convention (there are no Court decisions on this issue of the right of prisoners to marry and produce children, but a series of Commission decisions), the Court of Appeal also ruled that Article 12 did not offer an *unqualified* right to procreate. The case of *X v United Kingdom* 1975 suggested that a prisoner's ability to procreate 'falls under his own responsibility' and has not, as such, 'been denied by the State'. Moreover the restrictions in Article 8(2) have been taken to apply to rights under Article 12. The European Commission of Human Rights (1978) stated that:

> . . . an interference with family life that is justified under Article 8(2) cannot constitute a violation of Article 12.

Consequently, the restriction of conjugal access may be justified under Article 8(2) and this cannot be outflanked by a claim under Article 12.

In Mellor's case what was denied was not the *enjoyment of* conjugal rights, but the right to cement a newly formed family relationship by having children. The UK Court, drawing on the reasoning of the Commission, accepted that a prisoner excluded himself from the enjoyment of his rights, and that consequently the State could not be *required* to assist, at least on these facts, in the endeavour to produce a child.

Article 8(2) will not always, of course, offer such justification. If the proviso of Article 8(2) is to mean anything, then where it applies – under the doctrine of proportionality – there may be exceptional cases in which the interference with human rights is disproportionate. Such circumstances might include where, for medical reasons, the couple could not conceive naturally (such as low sperm motility, justifying the use of a procedure such as intracytoplasmic sperm injection (ICSI)), or where the woman's medical condition indicates that there is only a small window of opportunity left to the couple in which to conceive (e.g. medical deterioration of the womb, possibly after earlier miscarriages), so that conception would be unlikely after release from prison.

Hence, there are rights that come into play, although these do not lead the court to begin with the question of why it is that we should wish to deny the use of AIH, merely because someone is in prison. Answers to this question (beyond the notion that the denial is part of a punitive regime) are strangely unconvincing. These included 'serious and justified concern if prisoners continued to have the opportunity to conceive children while serving sentences'. Putting aside arguments about whether public concern is an appropriate touchstone for penal policy, why is the matter of concern and where is the evidence for this? According to the Court of Appeal, a policy 'which accorded to prisoners in general a right to beget children by artificial insemination would . . . raise difficult ethical questions and give rise to legitimate public concern'. It is true that matters of AHR do raise such problems, and that is one underlying rationale for the regulation of assisted conception under the 1990 Act. Yet AIH and even AID (artificial insemination by donor) are not regulated by the licensing provisions of the Act. The legislative view is that these procedures are not such that they require regulation in the public interest.

For those expecting radical change and the strong advancement of civil liberties, the Human Rights Act 1998 may prove a disappointment. We see from this case that there are areas of administration in which the judges will face questions of review and supervision with great caution, and radical change, if it were to come, will lie more in the political than the legal sphere.

'Not in front of the children?': procreative privacy, reproductive autonomy and a rose by any other donor; the 'right to know' argument

There may be more optimism for change through the courts and the use of the Human Rights Act 1998 in a challenge to one of the pivotal concepts of the Human Fertilisation and Embryology Act 1990, enshrined in Sections 31(4), (5) and (6). With effect from 2008, individuals may apply to the Register of Information that the Human Fertilisation and Embryology Authority (HFEA) is obliged to maintain about treatment services and children born of them. From that date 16-year-olds wishing to marry and, from 2010, 18-year-olds may apply to discover if they have been born following gamete donation. The HFEA must disclose if they hold any such information. As the law stands *the identity* of any gamete donor cannot be disclosed. A change to this law will require an amendment of the 1990 Act, unless current litigation forces an earlier review.

About 1 in 500 people in the UK is now born using donated gametes. In *Gaskin v United Kingdom* 1990, the European Court of Human Rights held that Article 8 of the European Convention on Human Rights, demanding respect for the private life of an individual, requires that 'everyone should be able to establish details of their identity as individual human beings'. This judgment was relied on in debate as the source of a right to know information about the genetic and personal identity of donors.

The HFEA may direct licence holders in fertility clinics to record information about the recipients of treatment, the services provided, and the identity of gamete donors and of any child subsequently born. If the licensee (the clinic) does not know whether a child has been born after treatment, this information must be stored for at least 50 years. The HFEA is required to keep a register of information acquired from licensed clinics, and gives an applicant aged over 18 the power to obtain specified and limited information, provided a 'suitable' opportunity for counselling is also made available.

There are four positions with regard to releasing information about gamete donation:

1. that no identifying information be provided
2. that identification may be made with the consent of the donor
3. that all identifying information be given
4. that some non-identifying information be provided.

The Act opts for the last of these positions. The precise form that this information is to take is unclear, because no regulations have been made. A late safeguard was written into the Act (by Section 31(5) which allows for regulations to be made; the safeguard could be withdrawn by the repeal of the Section but this seems unlikely), provided that the HFEA cannot be required to give information about the *identity* of a donor where that information was acquired before the HFEA could have been required by regulation to give the information. Thus even if *Regulations* are introduced allowing the disclosure of identifying information, those already born through assisted conception cannot benefit, without amendment of the 1990 Act, which the Government has announced it will not seek. A *Donor Information Consultation* paper, issued by the Department of Health in December 2001, reiterated this point, and has called for responses to its preliminary conclusion that, *if* any changes with respect to identifying information are to be contemplated, they should be confined to children born of future donation. This raises the issue about whether it is right that the provision of identifying information to offspring should be subject to a 'temporal' guillotine, with the effect that offspring born before the 1990 Act took effect can never access such information?

Interestingly, the Glover Report (1989) concluded that there should be a presumption that children born through semen donation should have access to knowledge of the identity of their biological fathers when they reach adulthood. As a result of worries about a consequent reduction in the supply of donors, the Report advocated a trial period of experiment following Swedish law. After the abolition of anonymity in Sweden (1984), there was an initial decline, not only in donors, but also in couples seeking donor insemination (DI) and physicians prepared to continue DI practice under the new decree (Law on Insemination' No 1140 of 20 December 1984, Article 4). Since then, in centres continuing to offer assistance, the numbers of donors have returned to their previous levels, although with two marked changes. Donors now tend to be older men, and also more often to be married men. The general experience, shared even by those who were most forceful in their opposition to the law, is that it has been successful.

The experience with adopted children seeking to discover their genetic identity is so strong that the denial of that interest to children of reproductive technology would be mistaken (see Braude et al., 1990; Haimes, 1990). The decision of what to tell donor offspring has long been one of the most problematic aspects of technological creation. The balance between preserving the identity of the donor and fracturing the identity of the resulting offspring has produced one of the deepest philosophical and pragmatic tensions.

Perhaps surprisingly, given the heat this issue generates, Golombok has reported that only 8.6 per cent of parents of children aged up to 12 have told the child of the DI, only 12 per cent of the mothers reported that they intended to tell their child some time in the future, whereas 75 per cent have decided not to do so. Yet over half of the women *had* told a friend or family member of the donation (Golombok et al., 2002).

In *Rose v Secretary of State for Health and HFEA* (2002) EWHC 1593 an adult, Joanna Rose and a six-year-old, EM, argued that a decision to withhold any information of their genetic origins was a breach of Article 8 of the ECHR. In a preliminary ruling Scott Baker J held that Article 8 was indeed engaged, if not yet on the evidence breached; that would be decided at a later hearing. He said it was clear from earlier cases that 'respect for private and family life requires that everyone should be able to establish details of their identity as individual human beings. ... A human being is a human being whatever the circumstances of his conception and an AID child is entitled to establish a picture of his identity as much as anyone else.'

Rights for life? The case of Zain Hashmi (2002)

Parents are often required to take difficult decisions. Indeed, framing and resolving issues on behalf of younger children might be thought to be a working definition of parenthood. Refusing a life-saving therapeutic opportunity for a child may be the most harrowing and troubling of any such decision. As the case of the conjoined twins Mary and Jodie (2000) amply demonstrated, it is a decision that we are publicly prepared to remove from parents *in extremis*. Having others take these decisions when the threat to life is chronic and not acute raises the clash of personal and social concerns more starkly than any other. This appears to be the position in which Raj and Shahman Hashmi – parents to 2-year-old Zain, born with thalassaemia-beta major – found themselves. (Thalassaemia-beta is a disorder that prevents efficient oxygen circulation through the blood supply, resulting in atrophied and then toxic tissue, which kills the sufferer.) Dr Simon Fischel of the Park Infertility Authority petitioned the HFEA on behalf of his patients to allow them to use assisted conception and embryo biopsy to establish a pregnancy and take stem cells from the umbilicus of any child subsequently born to Shahman Hashmi to establish cells for a bone marrow transplantation that would effectively save Zain's dwindling life. In December 2001, the HFEA announced approval of such genetic testing. Their decision was taken against the backdrop of the European Convention on Human Rights.

There are those who object to what they see as the 'designer' use of children, the 'mere' creation of a child to be used according to the specifications or benefit of another. Although this is not designing in the senses of choosing particular identifying features of the child for him- or herself, it *is* an instrumental use in the sense that embryos with the 'wrong' characteristics will be stored for use by others or allowed to perish. If correct, this is an objection that must be taken very seriously, although it does not prove decisive for everyone.

There may be an intuitive feel that, *if* this move from assisted conception to circumvent the consequences of infertility to the use of IVF techniques in therapeutic medicine – a form of therapeutic IVF – is to be sanctioned at all, then it should be permitted in a case such as the Hashmis. This represents a significant move – from assisted conception to conscripted conception. Unlike the embryo stem cell debate (still very much conducted in the realms of research possibilities), it seeks to put *in vitro* fertilization (IVF) and embryo biopsy to an immediate therapeutic use, which will involve not only making *use* of, but indeed *making*, an embryo and the child it may later become. Those who hold that an embryo *is* an individual like you and me object to this use. But even those who do not hold that view can distinguish between the instrumental use of an embryo for research and the *further* instrumental manufacture and use of a child, born from such an embryo, for the therapeutic benefit of another.

A further objection might be one of cruelty: to the ailing 2-year-old child and to his parents, even though apparently willing the procedure. For the stark fact is that the prospect of a successful outcome is not good. Dr Fischel put the possibility of successfully establishing a pregnancy after embryo creation and selection at 30 per cent, assuming that an embryonic match can be found. With a woman of Shahama Hashmi's age – she is 37 – this seems a generous call, although possibly within acceptable bounds. If the estimated chances of establishing a pregnancy successfully were much lower, say 15 or 20 per cent – would the HFEA's view be markedly, and appropriately, different? Or what if Shahama Hashmi were 47? Or 62? Should these factors affect our judgement? (See *R v Sheffield AHA ex parte Seale* 1994.)

The second issue for the HFEA was whether this treatment should be permitted in this type of case. By and large – and with the exception of marginal cases – the HFEA has avoided having to deal with cases involving access to assisted conception rather than treatment-type issues. It is a moot point whether we should replicate the adoption model in AHR and assess the suitability for parenting of hopeful treatment candidates. Presently, the HFE Act 1990 provides that, before admitting patients to assisted conception programmes, account must be taken of the 'welfare of any child who may be born as a result of the treatment . . . and of any other child who may be affected by the birth' (Section 13(5)).

Here, a number of issues arise. The Hashmis do not appear to have excluded the possibility of other potential children of their already large family. What they asked for was not gamete donation and treatment to establish a family, but to use their own gametes to preserve and enhance what they have through another assisted and managed birth. It is not as though the additional sibling for Zain would be *no more than* a means to an end, worthy though that end might be. That child would have as good a chance as any other child born into that family of being loved and raised for his or her own sake, as much as for what they have been able to help to achieve. Children conceived and born in such circumstances are – we expect – likely to be loved and valued no less highly – perhaps quite the opposite – than any other child. But the instrumentality of any birth is rightly a matter of concern to the HFEA.

What if what was needed was not placental blood but a whole organ for transplantation? What if Zain nevertheless dies because the transplant failed, and his yet-to-be-conceived sibling was 'blamed' for his death? And what if this would not be Mrs Hashmi's fifth but her tenth child, and the third conceived in such circumstances, earlier pregnancies having either miscarried or failed to produce a successful donation? Under the welfare principle of Section 13(5), how should the clinic give effect to Zain's existing siblings' wishes? And what if one of them objects?

Many will feel – intuitively – that it is wrong to deny the Hashmis the chance to save the life of their dying 2-year-old. Many would dread to find themselves in such a position. There is of course a danger, in assessing each of these difficult personal dilemmas on a 'case-by-case' basis, guided often by our intuitive desire to ameliorate or alleviate suffering, that we sacrifice the long view and gradually accept as natural what is now manifestly experimental. The danger is that in doing so we lose sight of what we should seek to preserve.

There is an additional dimension to cases such as that of the Hashmis that engages what has been called 'one of the most fundamental provisions' of the European Convention on Human Rights, Article 2, the 'right to life.' Article 2 is an 'absolute' right: it not only protects life – subject to the death penalty and other uses of 'lawful' force that cause death – it secures it too. Indeed the recent decision of the House of Lords, in the much reported case of Pretty (in *R v Director of Public Prosecutions ex parte Pretty* 2002), asserts this strongly in denying that a right to life could ever support its antithesis, a right to die. (Pretty then took her case to the European Court of Human Rights.) Article 2 imposes not just negative obligations on contracting states, it imposes positive obligations too. When coupled with robust decisions in recent years in the European Court of Human Rights on the scope of the Article, it does suggest the need for a stringent examination and evaluation in medical treatment cases where there is (1) an appropriate decision taken by a 'public body' (within the meaning of the Human Rights Act 1998) and (2) an identifiable 'victim' adversely affected by that decision in a causally related manner.

Article 2(1) provides that:

(1) Everyone's right to life shall be protected by law. No one shall be deprived of his life intentionally save in the execution of a sentence of a court following his conviction of a crime for which this penalty is provided by law.

In *R v Cambridge Health Authority, ex parte B (a minor)* 1995 (a case before the Human Rights Act), a father sought to obtain health care for his dying daughter, B. She had responded to treatment for a lymphoma, but had then been diagnosed with leukaemia that was progressing rapidly. A bone marrow transplantation from her younger sister was followed by a further relapse and it was apparent that the cancer was terminal. Her doctors advised that further treatment was contraindicated, advice her father sought to challenge clinically and legally. A second opinion put B's chances of survival somewhat higher, and her father then approached the health authority to fund a second bone marrow transplantation. Taking account of the clinical judgement, the nature of the treatment and the estimated chances of success, the health authority declined to fund the treatment and B's father sought judicial review of that decision.

The judgement of the lower court indicated the wider implications of the case:

Of all human rights, most people would accord the most precious place to the right to life itself. Sometimes public authorities . . . have the power of life and death – or at least to decide, as I find is the case here, whether a person otherwise facing certain death should, by means of all resources at the public body's disposal, be given the chance of life.

R v Cambridge Health Authority ex parte B 1995 (at 6)

According to Laws J in *R v Cambridge Health Authority* 1995, certain rights were not only part of the European Convention of Human Rights but could also be found in 'the substance of the English common law'. In concrete terms that meant that:

. . . the law requires that where a public body enjoys a discretion whose exercise may infringe such a right, it is not to be permitted to perpetrate any such infringement unless it can show a substantial objective justification on public interest grounds.

R v Cambridge Health Authority ex parte B 1995 (p. 12)

In relation to a fundamental right, such as the right to life, Laws J argued that there was no room to draw a distinction, as the health authority had sought to do, between acts and omissions of a public body that might lead to death. Although that position might be tenable in criminal law, the authority's decision about the allocation of public funds, while not a positive act that threatened B's life, was nevertheless one about resources without which B would certainly die. That decision had, to the health authority's knowledge, materially affected for the worse B's chances of life. He concluded that her right to life had been 'assaulted' by the decision, and accordingly that it could be justified only by showing 'substantial public interest grounds' (*R v Cambridge Health Authority ex parte B* 1995, p. 14).

Laws J found that the Cambridge Health Authority had taken into account only *medical* facts and had paid no attention to B's family's views about whether the proposed treatment should be provided or withheld. He also castigated the authority's lack of transparency.

Thus, the right to health care becomes in fact a *right to transparency* about the tragic choices being negotiated and goes to the heart of the patient's relationship with the health-care system at all levels. It is a component – a rather ignored one – of the person's *right to know*. It engages important political and civic values as much as philosophical and ethical principles.

However, the Court of Appeal dismissed Laws J's finding as to the involvement of the family in the decision-making process peremptorily, saying that it 'entirely fails to recognise the realities of the situation' (*R v Cambridge Health Authority ex parte B* 1995, p. 8). It criticized the judge's approach to the whole question of resources, saying that:

> While difficult and agonising judgments have to be made as to how a limited budget is best allocated to the maximum advantage of the maximum number of patients, it is not something that a health authority . . . can be fairly criticised for not advancing before the court.
>
> *R v Cambridge Health Authority ex parte B* 1995 (p. 9)

Since then the Court of Appeal has, if anything, driven the dagger of utilitarianism deeper into the back of rights and resources arguments, although it has singularly resisted giving it a final twist. The dagger may be bloodied but the corpus of rights has yet to give up the ghost. In a later case (*R v North West Lancashire Health Authority ex parte A, D and G* 1999), the court confirmed that a health authority is entitled to make choices between various claims and that those choices will be open only to a limited review by the courts. The court further held that the precise allocation and weighting of priorities were a matter for each authority, allowing for exceptions in 'exceptional circumstances', which the authority could leave undefined. However, an authority *is* obliged to: (1) assess accurately the nature and seriousness of each type of illness; (2) determine the effectiveness of various forms of treatment for it; and (3) give proper effect to that assessment and determination in the formulation and individual application of the policy.

Nevertheless, the European Court of Human Rights has continued to affirm, most recently in *Osman v UK* 2000 (Osman was invoked in the Diane Pretty case (see above) in support of the state's obligation to protect life) that there is a range of policy decisions relating to state resources where the 'margin of appreciation' for state activity will remain broad. How do these considerations apply in the case of Zain Hashmi, in which no clinician was required to act against his or her clinical judgement, and no question of state resources is immediately involved? The examination of the rationality of the decision of the HFEA, if challenged, would be concerned not just with Zain Hashmi's health but with his life.*

Had the HFEA refused a licence to carry out this procedure, could it have been claimed under Article 2 to cause the death of Zain (were it to happen) such as to have infringed his 'right to life'? It is clear from Article 2 jurisprudence that there must be a causal link between the death and the state's (failure to) act: *LCB v UK* 1998. In *Airedale NHS Trust v Bland* 1993 and *NHS Trust v M* 2001 (cases of withdrawing treatment, or hydration and nutrition), the Courts have held that death was caused not by the withdrawal (an *omission* to continue treatment and not a positive act) but by the underlying condition. The President of the Family Court, Dame Elizabeth Butler-Sloss, held that the distinction between acts and omissions identified in *Bland* as far as English law is concerned survives Article 2. She observed that:

> The phrase 'deprivation of life' must import a deliberate act, as opposed to an omission, by someone acting on behalf of the state which results in death
>
> . . . .

Article 2 therefore *imposes a positive obligation* to give life-sustaining treatment in circumstances where, *according to responsible medical opinion, such treatment is in the best interests of the patient* but does not impose an absolute obligation to treat if such treatment would be futile (emphasis added) (*NHS Trust v M* 2001).

---

*This decision was successfully challenged in December 2002, but permission was given to appeal.

Thus, it seems clear that:

- there will arise circumstances in medical law where Article 2 does indeed impose a positive obligation
- 'deprivation of life' must import a deliberate act, as opposed to an omission, by someone acting on behalf of the state which results in death
- *the positive obligation* to give life-sustaining treatment arises where, *according to responsible medical opinion, such treatment is in the best interests of the patient*; indeed, according to Cazalet J in *A NHS Trust v D* 2000 no Article 2 infringement is arguable where the treatment *is* in the best interests of the patient (as there, a decision *not* to treat the patient was in their best interests where there was a 'tragic irreversible worsening lung condition' such that their 'life span must be very short')
- nevertheless, 'there will be a range of policy decisions relating *inter alia* to the use of state resources, which it will be for [the State] to assess on the basis of their aims and priorities' (*Osman v UK* 2000).

So far, then, in this respect, we can say that:

- The HFEA is a public body within the Human Rights Act.
- If it had made a decision to refuse sanction for the proposed treatment, it would *not* have been comparable to withdrawing hydration and nutrition from a patient in a permanent vegetative state, such as Tony Bland. In that case, the House of Lords held that Bland would, if the treatment were withdrawn, die from the underlying acute insult, not from the omission to (continue to) act. In Zain Hashmi's case death would have resulted from the chronic congenital condition had the HFEA refused to sanction treatment (which has a 95 per cent chance of success once pregnancy is established).
- In other words, the HFEA would have prevented access to a therapeutic opportunity, which did not require state resources, where there was no threat to the *life* of others and, whatever the likelihood of the success or otherwise of the therapeutic treatment, where it was clear that *it was not futile*.
- The treatment was considered by his doctors – a responsible medical opinion – to be in his best interests.
- Although it is clear that there is no *positive right to demand medical treatment* (*R v Cambridge Health Authority ex parte* B 1995; *R v North West Lancashire AHA ex parte A, D and G* 1999), this was *not* a case immediately enjoining scarce state resources, such that the conflict entertained and discussed by the Court of Appeal in *ex parte B* applied.
- Indeed, this was a case that 'seriously affects the citizen's health' thus requiring substantial consideration by the HFEA, and careful scrutiny by the court as to the decision's rationality. ('Do not resuscitate'

policies (i.e. do nothing orders) have been felt to be sufficiently vulnerable to Article 2 challenge to lead the Department of Health to issue new guidance (HSC 2000/028).)

Denial would not have constituted a refusal of treatment that would merely have made life better (as in *A, D and G*), or that was beyond the clinic's resources (as in *ex parte B*), or that would be futile or not in the patient's best interests (as in *Airedale NHS Trust v Bland* 1993 and *NHS Trust v D* 2000), or would require the balancing of one right to life against another (as in *In Re A (Conjoined Twins)* 2000). It would have been the refusal of the HFEA for a treatment that would offer a chance of life.

The strongest ground for denial (and the one on which the HFEA was prepared to comment during its consideration) was the welfare of any child to be born for this heroic conception. This concerned the instrumentalism of the original 'conception' and also the possibility of that child in later years being called upon to be a 'donor' of blood for his or her brother. (To be successful as far as Zain is concerned, any such intervention would most likely have to be in his sibling's first 2 or 3 years of life.) Hence the HFEA came to weigh the 'welfare' of this (hypothetical) child against the claimed 'right to life' of Zain, the existing child.

Although *not* an exact analogy, there are echoes of the case of the conjoined twins (2000). In Mary's case there was no benefit to her of the operation to separate them because that operation would kill her. In that case the court balanced the interests of one against the other and in so doing chose 'the lesser of two evils'. Although each twin had a right to life, the court held that the *quality of that right* had to be a consideration. In Zain's case, like Jodie's, there is an expectation of a relatively normal life if the procedure is authorised. In Mary's case the operation would shorten her life. In *this* case, the 'operation' (to take a biopsy from an embryo, later to be implanted in the hope of leading to a successfully pregnancy) will not physically harm the resulting child. The question is whether the balance of any psychological harm to the child's welfare would be sufficient to offset any claim that Zain might have to a right to life or, more correctly, the chance of a hope to continue living. The HFEA decided that it was not, a decision that required both wisdom and courage, but one also influenced by the framing of right to life issues. It remains to be seen how influential such rights will prove upon the courts.

Reproductive rights: the next act

These cases and the possible scenarios that we have reviewed show the nature and breadth, the pace and the scope of the changes and challenges that the reproduction revolution has forced upon us. Recent high-profile examples of gay fathers, and parents of twins and triplets who found a surrogate to carry the pregnancy after a donated egg was fertilized with sperm provided by one of them, illustrate further possibilities to which 'reproductive rights' give rise. Taken together, these discrete examples illustrate how reproductive innovations:

- have the ability further to melt down previously understood elements of the nuclear family
- may engage what we might call 'cyber-reproduction' – or e-production (taking the 'r' out of reproduction) – with the presence and the promise of the internet
- can create a formidable array of new problems for public policy.

Such concerns lie at the heart of modern engagements between AHR and rights-based arguments and, rather than enabling the reproductive family to settle down and mature, they are likely to ensure continuing turbulent developments.

Table of cases

In Re A (Conjoined Twins) (2000) 4 All ER 961.
Airedale NHS Trust v Bland (1993) 1 AC 789.
Gaskin v United Kingdom (1990) 12 EHRR 36.
Hecht v Superior Court of the State of California (1993) 20 California Reporter 2d 275.
LCB v United Kingdom (1998) 27 EHRR 212.
MacFarlane and another v Tayside Health Board (1999) 4 All ER 961.
NHS Trust v D (2000) 2 FLR 677.
NHS Trust v M (2001) 2 WLR 942.
Osman v United Kingdom (2000) 29 EHRR 245.
Paton v Trustees of British Pregnancy Advice Service (1978) 2 All ER 987.
R v Cambridge Health Authority ex parte B (1995) 23 BMLR 1.
R v DPP ex parte Pretty (2002) 1 All ER 1.
R v Home Office ex parte Mellor (2001) Human Rights Law Report 38.
R v Lord Saville of Newdigate ex parte A (1999) 4 All ER 860.
R v North West Lancashire Health Authority ex parte A, D and G (1999) Lloyd's Rep. Med. 399.
R v Secretary of State for the Home Department ex parte Daly (2001) 2 WLR 1622.
R v Sheffield AHA ex parte Seale (1994) 25 BMLR 1.
Roe v Wade 410 US 113 (1972).
Rose and Another v Secretary of State for Health and HFEA (2002) EWHC 1593.
X v United Kingdom (1975) 2 DR 105.
X & Y v Switzerland (1978) 13 DR 105.

References

Braude P, Johnson MH, Aitken RJ (1990) Human fertilisation and embryology bill goes to report stage. Editorial. British Medical Journal 300: 1410–1412.

Department of Health (2001) Donor Information Consultation: Providing information about gamete or embryo donors. London: DoH

Dworkin R (1985) A Matter of Principle. Cambridge Mass: Harvard University Press.

Dworkin R (1993) Life's Dominion. London: Harper Collins.

Dworkin R (1996) Freedom's Law. Oxford: Oxford University Press.

Dworkin R (1997) Taking Rights Seriously. London: Duckworth.

Glover J (1989) Fertility and the Family. London: Fourth Estate.

Golombok S, Brewaeys MT, Giavazzi D, Guerra D, MacCallum F, Rust J (2002) The European Study of Assisted Reproduction Families: The transition to adolescence. Human reproduction. Cited in Department of Health (2001).

Haimes E (1990) Recreating the family? Policy considerations relating to the new reproductive technologies. In: McNeil M, Varcoe I, Yearley S (eds), The New Reproductive Technologies. London: Sage.

Hale B (1997) The Test Tube to the Coffin. Hamlyn Lectures, London: Stevens.

Harris J (1998) Rights and reproductive choice. In: Harris J, Holm S (eds), The Future of Human Reproduction. Oxford: Oxford University Press.

Robertson J (1994) Children of Choice: Freedom and the new reproductive technologies. Princeton, NJ: New Jersey University Press.

CHAPTER 5

Donor-assisted conception: what can we learn from adoption?

JULIA FEAST

The debate about whether or not the psychological tasks of parenting adopted children are comparable to parenting children who have been born as a result of donor-assisted conception is ongoing. The end of the twentieth century and the beginning of the twenty-first have seen a significant increase in children born as a result of donor-assisted conception. Traditional, ethical and moral boundaries are constantly being tested and challenged, and the discussion about the needs of the children born through such conception is long overdue. Medical advances have led to complicated family relationships, which need to be thought about within a social and ethical perspective. The subject of adoption has attracted a great deal of interest. It has been researched and much has been written about, giving professional and other people affected by adoption a greater insight into the dynamics of the adoption process. There have been lessons learnt about best practice to ensure that the needs of children and adults involved are not overlooked.

This chapter looks at the history of adoption from a UK perspective, in terms of the development of openness and how it now acknowledges the life-long needs of adopted people. It considers some of the similarities and differences in the issues and dilemmas faced by adoptive parents and parents of children born as a result of donor-assisted conception, and how these can best be managed without compromising the welfare of the child.

The history of adoption and the principle of openness

When adoption was first legalized in 1926, it was viewed primarily as a way of providing children for couples who were not able to have family of their own. It was largely an adult needs-led service, which at the time did not give a great deal of thought to what might be the life-long implications for the children involved. Adopting a baby or child was something that was often not openly celebrated but was usually shrouded in secrecy for all parties involved. There was a stigma attached, particularly for the birth mothers, because illegitimacy was socially unacceptable. Deceit and pretence were prevalent. Birth mothers would be sent to a mother and baby home until the child was born and return to their home town, often unable to tell anyone and grieve openly for the baby they had relinquished to adoption.

> When we arrived home, my mother started putting clothing away, talked about all the local gossip and asking what I would like for dinner? I couldn't believe what was happening. I became acutely aware that this was how it was, how it was going to be. 'My child' was forgotten, everyone was acting as though nothing had happened. Only the darkness of my bedroom allowed me to give vent to the terrible pain that was knotted inside me.
>
> Denise (in Coleman and Jenkins, 1998)

Adoptive parents were encouraged to pass the child off as their own genetic son or daughter, enabling the stigma of the child's illegitimacy and their own infertility to remain hidden. Indeed adoptive parents were given a clear message from professionals that it was a new start for the child and that their previous history and information about origins would not play a significant part in their growing-up years. There was no real understanding or discussion of the effect of adoption on all involved, especially little awareness that the adopted children and adults may want to find out about their origins.

Adoption formed a legal 'severance' between the family of origin and the new family, but for many adopted people this 'severance' did not represent how they felt nor did it satisfy their need for information. An information leaflet provided for adoptive parents in the 1950s describes this practice:

> . . . provided that he has not grown up with the idea that his adoptive parents do not love him, or that there is some mystery about his origins, he will not dwell unduly on these matters or want to get in touch with his natural parents.
>
> Standing Conference of Societies Registered for Adoption (1949).

But, as history has shown, that was not the case. For many adopted people there was a wish to have more detailed information about the family of origin, and for some also a wish to make contact with the birth family. Studies by McWhinnie (1967) and Triseliotis (1973) provided some important information about the needs of adopted people. Triseliotis's study confirmed the importance of adopted people having access to information and knowledge about their origins and background:

> The adoptees' quest for their origins was not a vindictive venture but an attempt to understand themselves and their situation better . . . the self per-ception of us all is partly based on what our parents and ancestors have been, going back many generations. Adoptees too, wish to base themselves not only on their adoptive parents, but also on what their original parents and forebears have been, going back many generations . . . no person should be cut off from his origins.
>
> Triseliotis (1973, p. 166)

The voice and views of adopted people were eventually recognized in Section 26 of the Children Act 1975 (subsequently Section 51, the Adoption Act 1976), when a provision was made for adopted people to access identifying information about their origins. Adopted people were given the right to obtain a copy of their original birth certificate which gave information about their original name, place of birth and their birth parents' name(s) and address(es) at the time of birth. It also gave the adopted person the right to apply to the court to find out which adoption agency placed them for adoption. This meant that they had the opportu-nity to access the agency's records, which often give more detailed background information about their origins and adoption.

So, for many years, as observed in a Government White Paper (Department of Health, 1993, pp. 4.19–4.20), adoption was often a secre-tive process. 'Adopted children were often not informed of their status and could be traumatised if they discovered it by accident. It was impossible or difficult for them to discover anything about their birth parent, or for birth parents to discover anything about their children after adoption. A good deal of progress has been made on those issues since the 1976 Act. It is sen-sible and humane to encourage an open approach, provided always that the prospects for a secure and successful adoption are not jeopardised.'

It took 50 years from the 1926 Adoption Act for the needs of adopted children to be acknowledged and addressed through legislation. Today, adoption is no longer a process that carries stigma or is shrouded in secre-cy. But how does the adoption experience relate to the situation of couples and individuals who have to depend on donor-assisted concep-tion in order to create the child that they long for? What are the similarities to and differences from adoption? What learning has been gained from adoption, in terms of a child's identity and information needs, that is relevant to children born as a result of donor-assisted conception. Should such children have the same rights to identifying information as their adopted counterparts? These are crucial questions that are now beginning to receive far more attention in the public arena. It is therefore an opportune time to consider the knowledge that has been gained from adoption practice in relation to the experiences of donor-conceived people and their parents.

Legislation and truth about origins

It is generally now accepted that adoption needs to be a child-centred service where the underlying principles of openness and honesty are embraced. However, for donor-conceived children this is not the case. In adoption, the developments in the practice and principles are supported within a legislative framework that acknowledges the welfare of the child as being paramount, as laid down in the Children Act 1989:

> (1) When a court determines any question with respect to the upbringing of a child; or the administration of a child's property or application of any income arising from it, the child's welfare shall be the court's paramount consideration.

For donor-conceived children their welfare is viewed not as paramount but as needing consideration as reported in the Human Fertilisation and Embryology Authority's Code of Practice (March 2001, Section 13(5)):

> Centres should take all reasonable steps to ensure that people seeking treatment and any children resulting from it have the best possible protection from harm to health. Before providing any woman with treatment, centres must also take account of the welfare of any child who may be born or who may be affected as a result of treatment.

Current adoption legislation allows for adopted people, on reaching the age of 18 years, to have access to identifying information held on the birth certificate. This gives them the opportunity to initiate a search for their birth family or their genetic parent should they so choose. The 1975 Act was retrospective, giving all adopted people the right to access information about their origins if they so wished. In consideration of the concerns expressed at the time, people who were adopted before 12 November 1975 and were not aware of their original name have to attend a counselling interview before the information contained in their birth certificate is released.

For those born as a result of donor-assisted conception, the 1990 Human Fertilisation and Embryology Act gives them the right to apply at the age of 16 years to the Human Fertilisation and Embryology Authority (HFEA), to ask whether a person they are proposing to marry is genetically related to them. It also allows anyone from the age of 18 to enquire whether they were born as a consequence of treatment services. No identifying information is permitted and, as the legislation is not retrospective, this opportunity applies only to those born after 1991. They have no other right to any information about their biological parentage.

Once a child has been adopted, the parents are issued with a new certificate, similar in appearance to a birth certificate but with a fundamental difference because it states that it is an adoption certificate. It has been described as a document of truth. There is no similar facility for children born as a result of donor-assisted conception and no official document that recognizes their status. So, for donor-conceived people, the long birth certificate could be seen as a document that provides false information because it indicates that the named father has a genetic relationship, which is usually not the case. The birth certificate has nothing on it to indicate that one of their parents is not genetically linked. Thus, the facts surrounding their origins can remain secret. With such fundamental differences in the legislative framework, it is perhaps not surprising that parents of donor-conceived people see the parenting task of talking openly and telling the children the truth about their origins as not the same as if their child were adopted.

The anomaly in the law means that different practices exist between adoption and donor-assisted reproduction. In the latter, there are safeguards in place to maintain secrecy and for the child's individual identity needs not to be addressed. But, is this right and is there now evidence to suggest that the child should be told about his or her origins? If so, it then raises issues about what information should be recorded and passed on to enable parents of donor-conceived children to be in a position to answer their son's or daughter's questions about their origins.

Identity and a child-centred approach

Adoption has taught us a great deal about the importance of identity and family connectedness. Over the years adoption practices have been refined so that children's needs are hopefully at the forefront and are not superseded by adults' needs. Such experience, research and knowledge can be used to inform other situations where a child's identity and origins are at stake.

Like adoption, the ethics relating to donor-assisted conception and the rights of the child versus those of the adult are highly charged; this is an emotive subject. People may hold very strong personal, religious and professional views about the rights and needs of all the parties involved, but it is important that we are able to think into the future about the implications of denying donor-conceived children and adults the right to the same information as adopted people. Condoning and endorsing practices that deny donor-conceived people and their families information that may be central to their sense of self and well-being must be questioned and challenged.

Current practices in donor-assisted conception are primarily led by adults' needs. Unlike adoption, they are not fundamentally child centred. It is not uncommon to see advertisements in the national press on a regular basis, which appear to refer to children as a commodity rather than as human beings with their own needs:

> Egg sharing is ingenious and harmless . . . it neatly brings together surplus and shortage.
>
> Highly innovative, ethical and good value for money and for our patients.
>
> Egg sharing is a gift from one woman who has suffered the pain of infertility to another.
>
> *Evening Standard* (June 1999)

These quotes suggest that little attention is given to the child and that creating a family by using assisted human reproduction is very much an adult-led service. This perhaps reflects the time when these discussions and decisions are taken; because the child is not yet created, it is perhaps harder to keep the imagined child's needs in clear view. It would appear that much needs to be done if the professionals involved in providing donor-assisted reproductive services are to ensure that the end result of gamete donation – a child who will grow up to have his or her own needs and rights – is not forgotten.

Similarities and differences and the importance of identity

Adoption has often been reported as being fundamentally different because, unlike donor-conceived children, adopted people have been given up or abandoned by their birth parent (Shenfield, 1994; Shenfield and Steele, 1997). This view is largely inaccurate. In the years before 1975, the majority of birth mothers reported feeling that they had no choice in the adoption decision. The social climate meant that unmarried mothers were frowned upon and there were no services to help them keep their babies. Many birth mothers relate how they had been told that if they really loved their babies they would hand them over to a childless couple who could offer the security a child needs:

> Lurking beneath the surface of many of the discussions between the mother and the 'professionals' was a pernicious double-bind. If you really love your child you will give him or her up for adoption; if you keep the child then that is proof that you do not sincerely have his or her best interests at heart and therefore you are not a fit person to care for the child.
>
> Howe et al. (1992, p. 65)

The following statement also echoes a common experience faced by most unmarried mothers in the 1940s, 1950s and 1960s:

> I was told I had nothing to offer the child that was to be born and that if I loved her I would give her up so that she could have a home and parents.
>
> Sorosky et al. (1978, p. 61)

Some suggest that the donation of gametes is a much colder action, which can leave the resulting child feeling devalued and abandoned, because their needs have not been considered in the process (Turner and Coyle, 2000). In contemporary adoption it is frequently the case that children have not been relinquished willingly but adopted because of state intervention after evidence of physical and emotional neglect and/or parental incapacity.

However, it has been argued that there are few similarities between adoption and donor-assisted conception (Shenfield and Steele, 1997). Most children are adopted by strangers with no genetic or social link. It is true that this is usually one fundamental and important difference. In donor-assisted conception, the child usually has a biological link to one parent. Quite often the mother is the 'natural' mother but the paternal parent has no biological link because sperm provided by a third party have been used. In some cases it could be a donated egg. However, does this fundamental difference of a partial genetic link alter what is in the best interests of the child in terms of secrets and denying identifying information about the child's other biological parent?

The evidence from adoption is that it is crucially important for children to have detailed and accurate information about their origins if they are to make sense of themselves (Triseliotis and Russell, 1984; Howe and Feast, 2000). Identity formation and having a complete sense of oneself is, however, a complex process. As Triseliotis (2000, p. 92) says:

> Genealogy, heritage and roots have been found to be essential ingredients to the formation of self and identity but not the only ones.

And that,

> The adopted person's family of origin and ancestry, race and ethnicity, represent only one aspect of social identity but nevertheless, a vital one that cannot be ignored.
>
> Triseliotis (2000, p. 84)

Identity is not only a question of biological roots but also a matter of nurture and the quality of relationships experienced in childhood. It is not just a single component that makes us who we are, and gives us our unique identities and individualism, but several, such as personal experience, social relationships, physical appearance, heritage and genes.

In adoption, the expectation is that adoptive parents will inform their children about their adoptive status and origins, giving their child the opportunity to seek information about their heritage and birth parents if they so wish. Should this be different for donor-conceived children because one of their parents is genetically related?

It could be argued that revealing the donor-conceived status to the child may not be in his or her best interest, particularly as, unlike adopted people, they cannot access identifying information to help them make sense of themselves. They cannot fill in the gaps they may be faced with in their genetic make-up, if and when their donor-conceived status is disclosed.

Perhaps the old saying 'what you never had you never miss' could apply. But several studies have shown that being truthful and honest with children about their origins:

> is central to their identity formation and their mental health. Evasiveness, secrecy and avoidance have been found to generate mistrust.
>
> Triseliotis (1973)

> Sharing such information with children is not, therefore, a matter of choice but an obligation on parents and substitute carers.
>
> Triseliotis (2000)

A few studies have looked at this issue. Most recently, a study by Turner and Coyle (2000) provides a particular insight into the needs of donor-conceived adults and the similarities they have with adopted people. They surveyed 16 donor-conceived adults between the ages of 26 and 55, and asked about identity experience, including the issue of secrecy and disclosure of their donor-conceived status. They also investigated their experience of trying to trace and search for their genetic father (the donor), their current perception of donor insemination, and how families should manage openness versus secrecy.

The authors reported that 'a consistent finding within the study was the negative and ongoing effects of withholding secrets and the knowledge that "things were not quite right", which supports previous research that found that secrecy in families is damaging and that children pick up hidden clues' (Karpel, 1980; McWhinnie, 1995). The following quotes taken from the study illustrate the participants' views and experiences:

I always felt like I didn't belong with these people – I searched for evidence of my 'adoption' for many years as a child. . . . It [the withholding of information] created a 'shroud of secrecy' and a 'sense of shame' about something I could sense but of what I had no real knowledge – I always had suspected something wasn't 'kosher' – but didn't know what it was – there's no way my sense of self esteem could not have been damaged by that experience.

Rachel (in Turner and Coyle, 2000, p. 2045)

Part of me was shaken and profoundly shocked. Part of me was utterly calm, as things suddenly fell into place, and I was faced with an immediate reappraisal of my own identity.

Imogen (in Turner and Coyle, 2000, p. 2044)

Implications of denying information

By its very nature, parenting children who are not genetically related presents different, difficult and extra challenges to the parenting task. It is easy to see how both adoptive parents and parents of donor-conceived children may wish to forget about the child's origins because it may be a constant reminder of their own infertility, something with which they may not have come to terms. Others may want to be open but find they cannot, and then struggle with the psychological and medical implications of not revealing a fundamental fact, which may have a profound effect on the decisions the donor-conceived or adopted person makes in his or her life. The evidence from studies undertaken in adoption is that being open and honest brings potential opportunities for both adopted and donor-conceived people (Triseliotis, 1973; Howe and Feast, 2000).

It seems that there is a lag in the consideration of psychosocial consequences of the new treatments. It is generally acknowledged how important it is for relationships to be built on a foundation of truth and trust. Technical progress should not therefore undermine society's knowledge base and the importance of having a moral and humane stance. In an era when the human genome project is opening up ever new possibilities, it would seem to be untenable that groups of individuals – children of donor gametes – be systematically denied access to information that may affect their physical and psychological well-being. To make informed life decisions, accurate information is a necessity. Without this, potential travesties will occur, e.g. not being able to access medical information that can fundamentally affect lives.

A poignant example was a case of a 53-year-old woman. She was attending her father's funeral when a cousin's husband came bounding up and informed her that they had something in common. She learnt for the first time that she was adopted. Although she tried to come to terms with this information and appreciated her parents' position in all of this, she could not help feeling resentful. She was married but had made a conscious decision not to have any children because her brother had died from a genetically inherited disease. The irony now for her was that he was not related and therefore she could have had the children she had longed for.

A similar example was reported last year. A 9-year-old donor-conceived child was discovered to have a potentially fatal condition known as Opitz's syndrome. It was subsequently learned that his genetic father carried this inherited single gene disorder. This sperm donor had fathered 43 babies from a London clinic each with a 50:50 chance of inheriting this rare disease (Rogers, 2001).

Knowing how crucial it can be to have accurate and updated family medical history, there is a case for becoming more proactive in informing the Government and legislators about the importance of people having access to information that may profoundly affect their future. To learn that you have a genetically inherited disease that could be cured with the assistance of someone related to you (such as leukaemia or kidney disease), but not be able to contact such a relative, must surely be wrong. In adoption there are channels available to help locate relatives in these circumstances. We need to question why donor-conceived people are discriminated against, because they are currently the only group of people whose need for information is not recognized.

Discovering the secret

One of the concerns of parents of donor-conceived children is that, if the child knows the circumstances of their conception, it could have a negative affect on the quality and strength of their relationship. However, the experiences from adoption have taught us that openness does not prevent the development of deep and lasting bonds. Most adopted people feel that their adoptive parents are their real parents. It may be more damaging to the parental relationship to discover later in life that they had not been told the truth about their origins. Unless nobody else knows about the origins of the child, be it adoption or donor-assisted conception, there is always a potential risk that the secret will be disclosed, possibly in distressing circumstances, such as a family argument or parental separation and divorce. Adopted people who discovered their adoption status in an unplanned way report how shocked they had felt and how difficult it was for them to come to terms with the idea that they had been living a lie. The following quote is from a donor-conceived adult but it could equally be from an adopted person who was told about his or her adoption late in life:

> I felt a considerable amount of regret about how utterly senseless it had been for my parents to keep this information [being a donor offspring] from me for so long. My mother expressed a fear that both of them felt during my childhood that if I had found out my dad was not my genetic father, I would have rejected *him*. The tragic irony of this was the sense of rejection I sensed from him [his emphasis] that there was something wrong with me that made him seem so distant from me.
>
> Peter (in Turner and Coyle, 2000, p. 2045)

> Being told that I had been conceived artificially using a stranger's sperm was like being hit by a train. It didn't hurt. I wasn't angry or grief stricken or excited. I felt annihilated. It felt as though I had been told something immensely important but meaningless: somehow, the most important thing I had ever been told was empty of content.
>
> Gollancz (2001)

For some, the discovery of the truth actually helped them make sense of things that had never felt quite right. The following echoes the experiences of both adopted and donor offspring adults, which clearly demonstrates how similar the feelings of a late discovery of a secret are:

> The secret which my own mother had carried for so many years was clearly a heavy burden and while she has never admitted to feelings of shame and guilt over her original decision to bear the child of a complete stranger, it was inevitable that the strain of keeping the pretence for so long would lead to resentment and frustration which eventually became focused on me. Little wonder that I felt confused both by my mother's attitude towards me and my own feelings of not fully belonging and a growing sense of ambiguity about my identity that I was not able to understand or articulate.
>
> Whipp (1998, donor-conceived individual)

I felt a mixture of shock and disbelief. I loved and trusted my parents but being told I was adopted the day before I got married had a devastating affect. Yet it was also a feeling of relief as it helped explain why I looked so different, why I was not so academically successful as my 'parents'. To some extent it helped me understand the feelings of difference that lay within me for as long as I can remember. The feelings I had were based on a reality.

Maureen (adopted person)

Openness and opportunities

Evidence is mounting that maintaining secrets and denying people important information about themselves can cause psychological damage, as illustrated in the examples above. Nevertheless, being open and honest and talking and telling is often one of the most difficult tasks for the adoptive parent. It also appears particularly difficult for the parents of donor-conceived people. It is a foregone expectation that adoptive parents will tell their children about their origins. Prospective adoptive parents have to show a willingness to tell the child about his or her adoption status and their attitude is reported to the court. Unlike parents of donor-conceived people, in adoption it is difficult to hide the truth about origins because it is recorded in an official way. For parents of donor-conceived people (particularly those born before a register was kept in 1991), it is a matter of choice. Arguably this creates a harder task for this group of parents who are required to make a very difficult decision themselves, often without long-term support or guidance.

The knowledge gained from adoption about the benefits of being open is extremely relevant to the current practices of donor-assisted reproduction. Unless this is given the attention it deserves, we are likely to be faced with a generation of people who have been denied the opportunity to access important information about themselves.

A recent Children's Society study about Adoption, Search and Reunion demonstrated that openness and telling are not always easy to implement (Howe and Feast, 2000). Yet these are considered essential tasks for adoptive parents if adopted people are to gain a true sense and understanding of 'self' and if their unique identities are embraced and valued. The authors studied 394 adult adopted people who searched for birth relatives (searchers) and 78 adult adopted people who had not searched but whose birth relatives had made an enquiry about them (non-searchers). They found that the majority of searchers (70 per cent) and non-searchers

(74 per cent) did not feel comfortable asking their adoptive parents for information about their birth family and their origins:

> Adoption was not talked about at all. I sensed my parents just didn't want to talk about it at all. They were just being protective toward me and . . . any questions that I asked they weren't always talked about. If I asked, they would just say, 'Well, you don't need to know about that' or they 'didn't know'.
>
> Angela (searcher, in Howe and Feast, 2000, p. 80)

> My parents didn't really want to discuss it with me any further when I asked for details, so when I was about nine or ten I rummaged through their bedroom and found various original birth certificates and court cases – the official papers for my adoption. . . . As long as I can remember I wanted to know more. My parents weren't very forthcoming when I spoke to them. They didn't want to divulge anything else about the adoption. I don't think they knew much though, to be honest. But they knew more than they told me, I've since found out.
>
> Jessica (non-searcher, in Howe and Feast, 2000, p. 78).

Although 40 per cent of adopted people said that their parents had been willing in principle to discuss the adoption and its background, it was not a subject they felt comfortable discussing.

> I always knew I was adopted. They were open that I was adopted but they never told me details – but then I never asked. I didn't like to ask . . . I just felt it was in the past and that's where it had to stay . . . . They also destroyed all the adoption papers as well, eventually. That was their way, you know, thinking it would never come up again.
>
> Martin (non-searcher, in Howe and Feast, 2000, p. 79)

> I've always known, as early as I can remember. My parents were as open insofar as they told us about being adopted and they had a little story book about how their children were adopted, how special we were that we were adopted but they didn't really talk about it as we got older. Our feelings about it weren't discussed. We didn't really know any information about ourselves. . . . It wasn't really discussed.
>
> Helen (searcher, in Howe and Feast, 2000, p. 76).

> I was five or six years when my parents told me I was adopted. . . . They must have done a good job of telling because I don't remember being upset or any negative feelings at all. I think I was made to feel quite special in a way. My father used to say 'you were chosen – we always wanted a girl'. I

> felt part of the family. I never felt different as such . . . I have very happy
> memories of my childhood.
>
> Liz (non-searcher, in Howe and Feast, 2000, p. 93)

The study highlighted how talking openly about the adoption and birth family was not an easy task for either the adopted person or the adoptive parent. The adopted people, although they may have wanted more information, were acutely aware of their adoptive parents' feelings and were keen not to cause upset by raising the subject:

> They always encouraged me to ask questions about my birth family and adoption but somehow I never felt comfortable asking. I felt I was being disloyal and was afraid that my parents would interpret it as that they were not good enough.
>
> Catherine (adopted person)

Although 'openness' and 'telling' are very much the principles that underpin adoption practice today, there is evidence that achieving this in practice continues to present challenges (Hundleby and Slade, 1999). However, adoptive parents are given opportunities to attend preparation groups and workshops where the wisdom of communicating openly with their child can be discussed. The experience of adopted people has taught us that being open about the adoption and the child's origins is not a one-off task but a subject that they may need to be revisited at various stages in the adopted person's lifespan (Howe and Feast, 2000).

The balance between acknowledging difference and a sense of belonging

Would-be parents often worry that openness about a child's origins might have a detrimental effect, because the child will automatically feel different. However, we know that, even when the fact that a child has no genetic relationship with his or her parent has been kept secret, the child can often sense a difference. Kirk's work (1964) highlighted the paradox of adoption. He brought into sharp focus the potential tension adoptive parents are faced with. On one hand, they are charged with the responsibility of integrating the child within their family, ensuring that the child is brought up with a sense of acceptance, belonging and sameness, while, on the other, they are expected to tell the child that he or she is adopted, which automatically creates a difference. Kirk argued that adopters who did not acknowledge difference and who 'rejected' difference were denying a relevant and potentially important aspect of their child's origins, sense of identity and worth.

Through openness and telling, differences can be acknowledged and valued. Unless this is achieved for donor-conceived children as well as for adopted people, there is a risk that the denial of differences from the non-biological parent may impact negatively on the child's self-esteem. Turner and Coyle's (2000) study included donor-conceived adults who had experienced this sense of difference. They found that, once the secret of the donor status had been disclosed, donor-conceived people had a better understanding of why they had experienced previously inexplicable feelings of difference throughout their lives.

Any parent is at risk of experiencing difficulties in loving and bonding with their children, in an unconditional way. How much more difficult it must be for the 'secret' non-biological parent to address and deal with when they are not able to acknowledge difficulties in terms of loving and bonding with a child who is genetically unrelated.

Roots, reasons and relationships

The findings from the Children's Society Adoption, Search and Reunion study (Howe and Feast, 2000) can be used to help reassure the 'social' parents of donor-conceived people that, although they are not genetically linked, this need not affect the development of affectional ties and bonding. The study showed that parenting and being the real Mum and Dad were not related to biological ties, but to do with the love and care given to the child over the years. Loyalty and feelings of love and affection were unhindered by the fact that they were not genetically related. This was also the case despite the finding that the process of telling and talking openly had not necessarily been easy. The study suggests therefore that telling does have benefits in that communication can be more open and offer reassurance on both sides:

> . . . even though my parents had always told me that I must never be afraid to ask them questions about my adoption and origins I knew from their body language that talking about it was not easy. In fact I also felt uncomfortable raising the subject as I felt that I was giving them a message that they were not good enough, which was certainly not the case. I love them dearly. But I must say that I take my hat off to my mum and dad as they were always open with me. They told me that they did find it difficult talking about my origins but this wasn't to be read by me that it should be a taboo subject. They reminded me that like anything in life practice makes perfect. We recognised it was an uncomfortable subject for us all. But my parents assured me that by communicating this, and by being frank and open with one another, we would be able to confront and understand the uncomfortable feelings. They told me that talking would eventually become easier

between us and feel better, and it did. When I decided to trace my birth family I felt I could do this knowing that deep down they understood how I felt and supported me. Talking about my birth to my adoptive parents no longer feels threatening or difficult. They know that I love them and I certainly know that they love me.

Rebecca

Parenting is not just about the genetic link. It is about being able to provide the child with love, security and being there at times when support is needed. For most adopted people the relationship established in childhood with adoptive parents remained strong and endured any subsequent relationships developed with the birth parents. The findings suggest that the relationships formed with 'social' parents during childhood therefore tend to be more robust and enduring than those based solely on biology.

The overwhelming need of most adopted people in the study was to find out more about three things:

• Why they were adopted (reason)
• Information about their own pre-placement history and background (roots)
• Information about their birth relatives, particularly their birth mother (relationships).

Adopted people in the study were asked to give their main reasons for seeking information from the adoption agency. The three main motivating factors to begin a search for information or birth relatives were:

1. To satisfy a long-standing curiosity about origins (82 per cent),
2. Needing to know more about oneself (77 per cent)
3. Need for background information (69 per cent).

When comparing this to the findings from Turner and Coyle's (2000) study, there are clearly many similarities. Donor-conceived adults also wanted to have access to basic background information about their roots, which may help explain what makes them who they are:

I'd like to know about my donor's health – half of my health history is missing and missed! I'd like to 'see' the personality traits I've inherited . . .

Rachel (in Turner and Coyle, 2000, p. 2046)

Howe and Feast's study showed that, whether or not the adoption was openly discussed, the majority of adopted people had thought about one or more of their birth relatives when growing up. Over 80 per cent of both searchers and non-searchers had wondered what their birth relatives looked like and whether they might look like them. Again, this was echoed in Turner and Coyle's study of donor-conceived adults:

> I needed to know whose face I was looking at in the mirror – I needed to know who I was and how I came to be – it was a very primal and unrelenting force which propelled the search and it was inescapable and undeniable.
> Rachel (in Turner and Coyle, 2000, p. 2046)

Howe and Feast's (2000) study compared the motivations behind a search for background information and contact with a birth relative for non-searchers and searchers. The study looked at feelings of difference and belonging; 50 per cent of searchers compared with 27 per cent of non-searchers described feeling different. The most common and glaring differences were physical dissimilarities:

> I looked different. I had a different personality and outlook.
>
> My character was different.
>
> I was more demonstrative.
> Howe and Feast (2000, p. 85)

However, feeling different and not belonging did not necessarily mean that the adopted person did not feel loved or feel positively about their adoption; 77 per cent of searchers felt loved by their adoptive mother compared with 91 per cent of non-searchers. With the adoptive fathers, 83 per cent of searchers and 89 per cent of non-searchers felt loved; 53 per cent of searchers and 74 per cent of non-searchers felt positive or very positive about their overall adoption experience. The adopted person's sense of feeling loved and belonging, different or the same, depends on a complex interplay of factors that need to be put in the context of the individual's adoption experience. The need to seek further information about one's background therefore cannot be simplified into categories of either being happily adopted or not.

Receiving information from the agency's adoption records had a powerful effect on adopted people; 65 per cent of searchers began to look for their birth mother immediately after receiving the necessary information. Within a 3-month period, 60 per cent had located their birth mother and in many cases this also meant that contact was established with other birth family members, such as siblings and grandparents. The majority of non-searchers (90 per cent) also agreed to have contact with the birth relative. Whether or not the contact with the birth relative was short-lived and difficult, or comfortable and long lasting, the majority of searchers (85 per cent) and non-searchers (72 per cent) described the reunion as being a positive experience. The research showed how the opportunity to receive information and perhaps have contact with a birth relative did answer important questions for the adopted person:

[It] Added a new depth and a sense of a perspective to my sense of identity.

[I] Feel more confident about myself.

[The] Process helped me understand myself.

I could make sense of the deep seated feeling of not belonging.

Over 80 per cent of both searchers and non-searchers said that the contact had answered important questions about their origins and background. Both searchers and non-searchers talked about feeling 'more complete as a person'. They had found the missing bits of their story:

Well, it's changed my personality. I'm more laid back now. I'm not so frustrated. I don't go off in a tantrum, because all the questions that were unanswered as a child and teenager and right up until my late thirties, things that have been going on in my mind, the questions that I've wanted to ask – its all been answered now . . . I'm at ease. I feel more at ease within myself for knowing. My [adoptive] parents say I'm not so uptight any more!

Susie (searcher, in Howe and Feast, 2000, p. 142)

Knowing that she wanted me. Knowing that she never forgot about me. To find things about my background and who I look like, that was the main thing . . . . It really worked out really well and we really get on. I think I'm very lucky.

Michelle (non-searcher, in Howe and Feast, 2000, p. 42)

For those who decided to have contact with their birth mother, 75 per cent of both searchers and non-searchers were still in contact with their birth mother after the first year. Five years on, 63 per cent of searchers versus 55 per cent of non-searchers were still in contact with their birth mothers.

The majority of the adopted people in the Howe and Feast (2000) study reported a positive experience of adoption. Originally, in adoption it was felt that, if a child had a strong sense of feeling loved and that they belonged, it would mean that the child would have no need to ask questions or sense a difference. The study seemed to confirm that human beings are complex, and love may not be enough to dampen natural curiosity and feelings of difference. For adopted people, the motivations for searching therefore seem a natural process to go through to help them understand themselves, and may similarly be a need for donor-conceived people.

There have, as yet, been few reports of donor-conceived individuals successfully finding and meeting birth relatives. If identifying information becomes available to donor-conceived individuals, they will have the same opportunities as adopted people to find out more about their genetic background and roots. The following quote is from a donor-conceived person who has found two half-siblings and his words powerfully bring into sharp focus the similarities in the feelings adopted people describe after a reunion experience:

> For me the discovery of these two has been like the warming of frozen soil after a hard winter, bringing growth and green into places that have seemed dead and desolate for 30 years and more. For all three of us, the delight we feel in each other's company and our certainty about the importance of our connection with each other, have a strength, immediacy and simplicity that is like a taste in the mouth: something known before and beyond the need for discussion. The meeting has brought me great joy and an even greater certainty about the need for an end to secrecy in DI.
>
> Gollancz (2001)

Managing the future and accessing appropriate services

As illustrated above, the evidence in support of the similarities between parenting an adopted child and a child born as a result of donor-assisted conception is strong. It seems essential, therefore, that the medical profession, and those who counsel would-be parents, take into account the potential life-long impact of this denial for donor-conceived children. The creation of a fertile egg followed by a birth, brings a human being who will have their unique needs and rights, including the right to have the opportunity to access information on their own identity:

> How could doctors . . . think that we wouldn't need or want some honest answers about our heritage? Without all this information, I will never feel complete.
>
> Verity (in Turner and Coyle, 2000)

It is important to let people who are creating families this way know that openness may be difficult and present challenges to the social parent, but that it does not necessarily adversely affect the quality of relationship.

As most adoptive parents agree, parenting a child who is not genetically related brings additional tasks to the nurturing and growing-up process. Consequently, it is important that prospective parents of a donor-conceived child should have access to services similar to those provided for adoptive parents, such as workshops to assist them in telling and being open about their child's background. We have to ask ourselves why adoption and donor-assisted reproduction are treated differently, and whether donor-assisted reproduction requires the same safeguards, standards and principles to make it a child-centred practice.

Equally, we need to pay attention to the long-term implications of being a donor. Adoption studies have reported the feelings of loss and grief that many birth mothers have suffered as a result of relinquishing their child for adoption (Bouchier et al., 1991; Howe et al., 1992; Wells, 1993; Hughes and Logan, 1993). Who is to say that for women who have donated eggs, some may not also experience feelings of loss and sadness? For example, the advertisement previously cited (*Evening Standard*, June 1999) encourages women experiencing fertility problems to donate their eggs in exchange for free fertility treatment. Situations may arise where the egg donor fails to become pregnant, whereas the recipient succeeds in becoming pregnant and may go on to experience feelings similar to birth mothers of adopted children.

Below are some suggested guidelines of how the needs of all involved in donor-assisted conception might be addressed:

- Need for legislation, which allows donor-conceived people access to identifying information about their donors.
- Ethically and morally there is a need for people to grow up in the knowledge of their origins, rather than being faced with a situation where they have to accommodate the shock and trauma of an unplanned disclosure.
- Access to counselling and information services. Such provision can help prepare prospective parents, both donors and the recipients of the implications, not only for themselves but also for the subsequent children born as a result of donor-assisted reproduction.
- Information about self-help groups, such as the Donor Conception Network, should be available so that prospective parents and parents of donor-conceived people have an opportunity to share and learn from their experiences.
- Need to prepare parents of donor-conceived children about the detrimental effects lack of disclosure/secrecy can have on family relationships.
- Need to acknowledge that, similar to adoptive parents, parents of donor-conceived children have additional tasks. The experience of

adopted people as well as the limited information so far available from donor-conceived children and adults shows that they have the capacity to accommodate information about their origins.

- Preparations for how to deal with difference, valuing it as well as engendering a sense of belonging.
- In setting up services for fertility treatment provision, there needs to be talking and telling workshops for parents, to increase parent's confidence and ability to be open about their child's donor-conceived status.
- Need for opportunities for health professionals such as doctors, nurses and counsellors working in fertility to access existing knowledge about the importance of information relating to a person's identity and heritage.
- Need for a range of counselling and information services to be made available to people who discover or are informed of their donor-conceived status.

Conclusion

One of the greatest challenges in life is parenthood. The ultimate goal is to provide a nurturing, loving and trusting environment so that children can grow up to become confident and secure adults and have the information necessary to make informed decisions. Until the shroud of secrecy that currently surrounds donor-assisted conception is lifted, the stigma attached to infertility and the feeling that it is something to be ashamed of may be perpetuated. We as a society therefore need to remove the barriers that currently exist for donor-conceived children, young people and adults, to ensure that everyone has the right to self-discovery and genetic connectedness. Recent research into adopted people's experience offers a rich source of material, indicating that parallels between people who are adopted and those born after donor-assisted conception should not be ignored. Ethically and morally there is a need for people to grow up knowing their origins, rather than being faced with a situation where they have to accommodate the shock and trauma of an unplanned disclosure. The learning from adoption practice is extremely relevant. If used and transferred to the area of donor-assisted reproduction, it will assist in developing an adult service that does not ignore the needs and rights of donor-conceived people.

References

Bouchier P, Lambert L, Triseliotis J (1991) Parting with a Child for Adoption: The mother's perspective. London: BAAF.

Coleman K, Jenkins E (1998) Elephants Never Forget: Reunions between birth parents and adoptees. United Kingdom: Signature Publications.

Department of Health (1993) White Paper Adoption: The future. London: HMSO.

Evening Standard (1999) (advertisement for egg donation), 29th June.

Gollancz D (2001) Donor insemination: a question of rights. Human Fertility 4(3): 164–167.

Howe D, Feast J (2000) Adoption, Search and Reunion: The long term experience of adopted adults. London: The Children's Society.

Howe D, Sawbridge P, Hinings D (1992) Half a Million Women: Mothers who lose their children by adoption. London: Penguin Books (now available and published by the Post Adoption Centre, Torriano Mews, London).

Hughes B, Logan J (1993) The Hidden Dimension. Mental Health Foundation.

Hundleby M, Slade J (1999) Project 16–18. Nottingham: Catholic Children's Society.

Karpel M (1980) Family secrets. Family Process 19: 295–306.

Kirk H (1964) Shared Fate: A theory of adoption and mental health. New York: Free Press.

McWhinnie AM (1967) Adopted Children: How they grow. London: Routledge & Kegan Paul.

McWhinnie AM (1995) A study of parenting of IVF and DI children: the social and legal dilemmas. International Journal of Medicine and the Law 14: 501–508.

Rogers L (2001) Sperm donor children may have fatal gene. Sunday Times 23 September.

Shenfield F (1994) Filiation in assisted reproduction: potential conflicts and legal implications. Human Reproduction 9: 1348–1356.

Shenfield F, Steele SJ (1997) What are the effects of anonymity and secrecy on the welfare of the child in gamete donation? Human Reproduction 12: 392–395.

Sorosky A, Baran A, Pannor R (1978) The Adoption Triangle. New York: Anchor Press/Doubleday.

Standing Conference of Societies Registered for Adoption (1949) What shall we tell our adopted child? Standing Conference of Societies Registered for Adoption.

Triseliotis J (1973) In Search of Origins: The experience of adopted people. London: Routledge & Kegan Paul.

Triseliotis J (2000) Treacher A, Katz I (eds), Identity Formation and the Adopted Person Revisited: The dynamics of adoption social and personal perspectives. London: Jessica Kingsley.

Triseliotis J, Russell J (1984) Hard to Place: The outcomes of adoption and residential care. London: Gower.

Turner AJ, Coyle A (2000) What does it mean to be a donor offspring? The identity experiences of adults conceived by donor insemination and the implications for counselling and therapy. Human Reproduction 15: 2041–2051.

Wells S (1993) Post-traumatic stress disorder in birth mothers. Adoption and Fostering 17(2): 30–32.

Whipp C (1998) Comparisons between the perspectives of adoptees and donor offspring, the forgotten foundlings of the reproductive revolution. Paper presented at the South East Post Adoption Network's conference entitled Are we creating children for parents? Are we ignoring the child's identity and genetic needs?

CHAPTER 6

Children raised in assisted human reproduction families: the evidence

CLARE MURRAY

The birth of the first *in vitro* fertilization (IVF) baby in 1978 (Steptoe and Edwards, 1978) marked a breakthrough in the development of assisted human reproductive (AHR) techniques, and new types of families that had not previously existed began to emerge. These families may be characterized by the degree of genetic relatedness between parents and their children, e.g. with IVF and the more recently developed intracytoplasmic sperm injection (ICSI) procedure, where the mother's egg and the father's sperm are used, the child is genetically related to both parents. Children conceived by donor insemination (DI) are genetically related to the mother, but not the father, and with egg donation (ED) the child is genetically related to the father but not the mother. When both a donated egg and sperm are used, as in embryo donation, the child is genetically unrelated to either parent. A child born through surrogacy may be genetically related to one, both or neither parents, depending on whether the egg, sperm or both gametes have been donated. Increased availability of AHR techniques has led to the creation of other types of family, arising from the growing number of single heterosexual women and lesbian women who are choosing DI to help them conceive a child, not because they have infertility problems, but because they wish to have a child without the involvement of a male partner. In these families, children are raised from birth without a father and in many lesbian families children grow up with two mothers. This chapter presents findings from research on parenting and the psychological well-being of children raised in these various family forms.

AHR families

What are the major concerns?

From a psychological perspective, a number of concerns have been expressed relating to the potential negative impact of assisted reproductive techniques on children's social and emotional well-being. One of the most hotly contested of these concerns has been whether or not children should be informed about the way in which they were conceived, particularly when this has involved the use of a donated egg and/or sperm. Donor insemination is the oldest assisted reproductive technique, with the first documented case appearing in the late 1880s (Achilles, 1992). Since its inception, secrecy has been an intrinsic feature of the procedure, with even the recipient woman in this case not being informed of the use of the donor sperm (Nachtigall, 1993). During the 1970s and 1980s, when the use of DI and egg donation became more widespread, it was common practice for clinicians to advise couples who were undergoing treatment that there was no need for the child to know about their donor origins (Mahlstedt and Greenfield, 1989). Today, DI is still cloaked in secrecy, and most children resulting from gamete donation grow up unaware that their mother or father is not their genetic parent. However, there has been increasing concern about the possible adverse effects of non-disclosure on family relationships and children's psychological well-being, reflected by a current trend among health professionals and social policy-makers in the UK and a number of other countries, such as New Zealand, to advocate openness as best practice in gamete donation families. Moreover, increasing public awareness of these issues has led to the emergence of parent support groups with the sole purpose of promoting the sharing of information with children conceived by donated gametes. Despite the moves toward encouraging openness, however, the identity of gamete donors in the UK and many other European countries remains protected by law.

The arguments for and against disclosure have been well documented in the literature, with proponents of each stance citing the benefits to the parents, parent–child relationships and the child's psychological development (Snowden et al., 1983; Snowden, 1990; Daniels, 1995; Shenfield and Steele, 1997; Walker and Broderick, 1999). Much of the evidence cited by those in favour of disclosure in gamete donation families has been extrapolated from adoption research and the family therapy literature. Findings from studies of adopted families consistently show that adopted children benefit from knowledge about their biological parents, and those children not given such information are more at risk for emotional problems and confusion about their identity (Triseliotis, 1973; Hoopes, 1990; Schechter and Bertocci, 1990). Similarly, it has been argued that donor conception children who are denied knowledge of, or information about, their donor are more likely to experience difficulties (Snowden, 1990; Baran and Pannor, 1993; Daniels and Taylor, 1993; Landau, 1998). However, doubts have been raised about the viability of the adoption model to explain the experiences of gamete donation children. These children are different to adopted children in that they have not been given up by their birth parents and, in most cases, are genetically related to one parent (Shenfield, 1994). In the case of egg donation and embryo donation, the child's mother is also the birth mother so these children have an additional biological link to their non-genetic parent (Shenfield and Steele, 1997).

Within the family therapy literature, it is widely acknowledged that secrets in families can cause tension and can threaten the harmony of family relationships (Bok, 1982; Clamar, 1989; Papp, 1993). It has been argued that children may become aware that information is being withheld from them, become anxious themselves and, in some cases, develop psychological problems. However, it is not clear whether this holds true for gamete donation children; it is not known, for example, whether these children are aware that information is being kept from them about their conception and, if so, whether this has a detrimental effect on their psychological well-being. It has also been suggested that parents, particularly fathers in DI families, may feel and/or behave differently towards a non-genetic child than a child who is genetically related to them, which may have an insidious effect on the child's sense of belonging and psychological well-being (Baran and Pannor, 1993). Other advocates of disclosure have argued that the child has a right to know the identity of his or her donor, using an interpretation of Article 7 ('the right to know one's parents') of the United Nation's Convention on the Rights of the Child 1989 (Daniels, 1995) and, more recently, Article 8 ('the right to respect for privacy and family life') of the European Convention on Human Rights (Human Rights Act 1998; Dyer, 2000), as justification for their position.

On the other hand, it has been argued that non-disclosure to gamete donation children protects both the couple and the child from existing negative societal attitudes about gamete donation, particularly DI and, more generally, about male infertility (Nachtigall et al., 1997). It has also been suggested that the relationship between the non-genetic parent and the child and the child's psychological health may be at risk if information about the donor conception were disclosed to the child, especially when no detailed information about the donor is available. These authors argue that parents should have the right to privacy and that it is their prerogative to keep information about their child's conception confidential should they choose to do so (Walker and Broderick, 1999).

Other concerns that have been expressed about the use of AHR techniques and the implications for family relationships and children's psychological functioning are related to the possible negative effects of the parents' experience of infertility, particularly, of having to undergo protracted infertility investigations and treatment. For some couples, the stress of infertility together with the stressful nature of the treatment procedures can have an adverse effect on their relationship (Cook et al., 1989). Where these relationship difficulties persist, problems may be more likely to arise for the child (Cox et al., 1989; Howes and Markman, 1989). It has also been suggested that, even after treatment has been successful, some parents continue to have problems coming to terms with their infertility and may experience difficulties in relating to their children (Burns, 1990). Other authors have argued that some parents who had problems conceiving may be more likely to emotionally over-invest, be over-protective, or to have unrealistic expectations of the child for whom they have waited so long (Burns, 1990; McMahon et al., 1995; van Balen, 1998). The social context of AHR families is also important and may influence family functioning, e.g. despite increasing public awareness and media coverage of infertility and infertility-related issues over the past decade, negative societal attitudes continue to surround the use of certain AHR techniques, particularly those involving a donated gamete (Klock, 1993). Consequently, families with a child created in this way are more likely to attract negative reactions from society in general as well as from other family members and friends.

These concerns notwithstanding, it is widely acknowledged within the psychological literature that children's healthy social and emotional development is fostered within the context of the child's attachment relationship with his or her parents (Bowlby, 1969, 1973; Main et al., 1985). According to attachment theory, how parents respond to their child is more important than genetic relatedness for the development of secure attachment relationships between parents and their children (Grossmann et al., 1985). This view is further confirmed by findings from research on families with children adopted in infancy, which show no difference between adopted and non-adopted children in the percentage of children who are securely attached to their mother (Singer et al., 1985). From this perspective, a child conceived by gamete donation would be expected to experience social and emotional problems only to the extent that a lack of a genetic tie with one or both parents has a negative impact on the security of the child's attachment relationship with his or her parents, either as a result of the parental non-disclosure about the child's conception or because the parents feel and/or behave differently towards a non-genetic child than to a child who is genetically related to them. In addition, it has been argued that specific parenting styles can exert a positive influence on children's social and emotional development, e.g. Baumrind (1989) found evidence to suggest that an authoritative parenting style, characterized by a combination of warmth and discipline, has a positive impact on children's psychological well-being. If non-genetic parents are no different to genetic parents with regard to parenting factors such as warmth and control, gamete donation children would not necessarily be expected to demonstrate more difficulties than children who are genetically related to their parents.

What does the research show?

Despite the concerns expressed about the potential negative outcomes for AHR parents and their children, there has, until recently, been an absence of empirical work to confirm or refute these views. In the first systematic longitudinal study of the consequences for these families, the European Study of Assisted Reproduction Families (Golombok et al., 1995, 1996, 2001, 2002a, 2002b) set out to assess the quality of parenting and the social and emotional development of the children in families created by the two most widely practised AHR techniques, IVF and DI, in comparison with families with a child conceived without any medical intervention (naturally conceived families) and adopted families.

The first phase of the study involved the collection of data from matched, representative samples in the UK of 41 families with a child conceived by IVF and 45 families with a child conceived by DI, and comparison groups of 43 naturally conceived families and 55 families with a child adopted in the first 6 months of life. At this stage, all the children were aged between 4 and 8 years (Golombok et al., 1995). All mothers were administered a standardized interview designed to assess the quality of parenting in these families, a modified version of the procedure developed by Quinton and Rutter (1988). Four overall ratings of quality of parenting were made based on information obtained over the course of the entire interview:

1. Mother's warmth towards the child.
2. Mother's emotional involvement with the child.
3. Mother–child interaction.
4. Father–child interaction.

In addition, both mothers and fathers were administered a standardized questionnaire assessing their perceptions of the degree of stress associated with parenting.

The social and emotional development of the children was measured with a standardized questionnaire designed to assess the presence of behavioural and emotional problems, completed by the child's mother and teacher. Measures of developing self-esteem and feelings towards parents were also administered to the child.

With regard to family functioning, the findings demonstrated that families with a child conceived by assisted reproduction (IVF and DI) obtained significantly higher scores on each of the overall ratings of quality of parenting in the above list. The quality of parenting in adoptive families fell between the assisted reproduction and the naturally conceived families. Consistent with this pattern of results, parents who had conceived a child without medical assistance reported significantly greater levels of stress associated with parenting. No group differences were found for any measures of children's psychological functioning, indicating that children in all groups were generally functioning well. Thus, the quality of parenting in families with a child conceived by IVF and DI appears to be superior to that demonstrated by families where no medical intervention (naturally conceived families) was required, suggesting that a strong desire for parenthood is a better predictor of family functioning than genetic ties between the parents and the child.

To increase the sample size and assess the potential impact of culturally prescribed attitudes towards assisted reproduction on the functioning of these families, identical procedures to those employed in the UK were used to obtain data from families in the Netherlands, Italy and Spain. Once these additional countries had been included, the total number of IVF, DI, adopted and naturally conceived families, respectively, was 116, 111, 115 and 120. The results from this larger study confirmed those of the original investigation (Golombok et al., 1996), indicating that the quality of parenting in families where a child had been conceived by assisted conception, irrespective of the use of donor sperm, was higher than that found in families where the child had been conceived in the usual way. Once again, no group differences were found for the psychological well-being of the children. The findings relating to the pattern of disclosure in donor insemination families are presented below.

More recently, a cohort of 21 families with a child conceived by egg donation has been recruited in the UK, allowing a comparison to be made between families where the child is genetically related to the father, but not the mother (egg donation families), and families where the child is genetically related to the mother, but not the father (DI families) (Golombok et al., 1999). At the time of the original investigation, these children were too young to participate because the practice of egg donation was introduced only in 1983 (Lutjen et al., 1984). The only significant difference found between these two family types was that parents of egg donation children reported less stress associated with parenting than mothers and fathers of a DI child.

Based on the results of these studies, it seems that early school-age children conceived by IVF, DI and egg donation experience warm, loving relationships with their parents, and are no more at risk for emotional and behavioural problems than children conceived without medical intervention. Such findings are consistent with those reported elsewhere in the literature of the quality of parenting and the psychological well-being of children in DI families (Kovacs et al., 1993), egg donation families (Soderstrom-Antilla et al., 1998) and IVF families, where different methodological approaches, comparison groups and measurement techniques have been employed: in France (Raoul-Duval et al., 1993), Belgium (Colpin et al., 1995), the Netherlands (Van Balen, 1996), the UK (Weaver et al., 1993; Papaligouras, 1998) and Australia (McMahon et al., 1997). Furthermore, there is no existing evidence to suggest that IVF, DI and egg donation children are at risk for cognitive impairment (Mushin et al., 1986; Yovich et al., 1986; Morin et al., 1989; Brandes et al., 1992; Raoul-Duval et al., 1993; Ron-El et al., 1994; Cederblad et al., 1996; Olivennes et al., 1997; Gibson et al., 1998; Levy-Schiff et al., 1998).

In the UK, the families were followed up as the children approached adolescence (Golombok et al., 2001): 34 of the original IVF families, 49 of the adoptive families and 38 of the families where the child had been conceived naturally were assessed as near as possible to the child's twelfth birthday. The response rate for IVF, adopted and naturally conceived families, respectively, was 87, 89 and 97 per cent, excluding those who could not be traced. Mothers, fathers and children were administered a combination of standardized interviews and questionnaires to assess two aspects of parenting thought to be important for adolescents' psychological well-being – warmth and control. It was found that, in general, IVF parents continued to experience positive relationships with their children. Both IVF and adopted mothers, however, were found to be less sensitive towards their child, and their children reported them as less likely to engage in reasoning during disputes. Thus, any differences found between the mothers appeared to be related to the experience of infertility, rather than IVF in itself. In spite of these differences, the IVF and adopted children regarded their mothers as more dependable than did naturally conceived children. With regard to the psychological adjustment of the children, IVF children at age 12 were found to be functioning well (Golombok et al., 2001).

The UK DI families were also assessed as the children reached adolescence (Golombok et al., 2002a). This is a time when, for many children, identity issues become more prominent. Research on adoptive families has shown that, as they pass through the transition into adolescence, adopted children show higher levels of behavioural problems than their non-adopted counterparts (Maughan and Pickles, 1990; Miller et al., 2000), as well as an increased interest in their biological parents (Hoopes, 1990). To the extent that DI children are thought to resemble adopted children, a similar pattern of findings would be expected in DI families.

Of the DI families, 37 were compared with the 49 adopted families and a new group of 91 families who had conceived a child spontaneously after experiencing a period of infertility, in order to control for the desire for a child. Employing the same measures and procedures described above (Golombok et al., 2001), the results revealed that DI mothers demonstrated higher levels of warmth towards their children than mothers from the other two groups. DI fathers were less likely to become involved in serious disputes with their children, and less likely to reason with their child when conflict did occur. It may be the case that the lack of a genetic link between DI fathers and their child makes these men feel less interest in, or less right to being involved in, the discipline of their child. Although the results may support the view that DI fathers are more distant from their children, it must be borne in mind that the data obtained from children themselves did not reflect this pattern of findings. Moreover, DI fathers showed just as much warmth to their child as the other fathers. With regard to the socioemotional development of the children, no group differences were found, showing that DI children at age 12 continue to function well.

The families from the other European families were also followed up when the children were 12 years old (Golombok et al., 2002b): 102 of the IVF families, 94 of the DI families, 102 of the adopted families and 102 of the families with a child conceived naturally were assessed, and a similar pattern of findings was found with regard to the quality of parent–child relationships. Where differences between the groups were identified, these tended to reflect more positive functioning in the AHR (IVF and DI) families, except for a small proportion of IVF and DI mothers and fathers who were found to be over-involved with their child. The IVF and DI children did not differ from the adoptive or naturally conceived children with respect to psychological adjustment.

Thus, the evidence to date suggests that the fears about the potential negative effects on the quality of parenting and the psychological development of children in families created by AHR (i.e. IVF, DI and egg donation) are largely unfounded – both parents and children appear to be functioning well. This remains the case during the transition from childhood to adolescence, when increased difficulties might be expected for these children and their parents.

It is important to note, however, that certain methodological limitations, such as low response rates and small sample sizes, are common to many studies of assisted conception parents and their children, highlighting the need for ongoing systematic investigation of these families. With regard to other, more recent, AHR techniques (i.e. ICSI, surrogacy and embryo donation), no study has yet assessed the quality of parenting and the socioemotional development of children in families created by these techniques.

Gamete donation families

Pattern of disclosure, parents' decision-making processes and the psychological impact on the child

As previously noted, the issue of whether or not to tell children about their donor origins has been the subject of much debate. Most of the research on the pattern of disclosure in gamete donation families has tended to focus on DI families, possibly because this is the oldest and most widely practised of the gamete donation procedures.

In the first phase of the European Study of Assisted Reproductive Families (Cook et al., 1995) British mothers of 4- to 8-year-old children conceived using DI were interviewed about their attitudes towards disclosure about the nature of their child's conception. Systematic information was obtained from the mothers about whether or not they had told their child about his or her donor origins and whether or not they had told any family members or friends. Mothers were then asked about the reasons for their decision. Remarkably, the results showed that not one of the 45 sets of parents had told their child about the way in which he or she had been conceived, preferring instead to have their child believe that their social father was also their genetic father. Almost all the mothers (80 per cent) reported that they had no intention of telling their child in the future, 16 per cent were undecided and only 4 per cent planned to tell their child at a later stage. Despite choosing not to disclose to their child about their donor origins, almost half of the DI parents had told a friend or family member, creating a real possibility that the child would find out from another source. When asked to elaborate on their decision for their non-disclosure to their child, the mothers cited one or more of the following reasons:

1. To protect their child from what they believed would be the potentially devastating effect of finding out that the man they know as their father is not their genetic father.
2. To protect the father from both possible rejection by the child and from other people learning about his infertility.

3. As a result of lack of information on when, how and what to tell their child.

The same information was obtained from DI mothers in The Netherlands, Spain and Italy (Golombok et al., 1996), and an identical pattern of findings emerged: not one set of the 111 DI parents had told their child about the way in which he or she had been conceived, and most (75 per cent) had no plans to tell their child in the future. Interestingly, Italian parents were most against telling, with 100 per cent having decided never to tell, followed by the UK (80 per cent) and Dutch parents (75 per cent). Spanish parents appeared to be more flexible about the possibility of disclosing information to their child, with only 48 per cent reporting that they were definitely never going to tell. In line with the findings from the UK study, nearly half the DI parents had told a friend or family member about their child's donor origins. Analysis of the decision-making process of the Dutch DI parents revealed a similar picture to that found in the original study; the large majority of parents (82 per cent) attributed their non-disclosure to a desire to protect their child and 30 per cent of parents reported a desire to protect the father–child relationship (Brewaeys et al., 1997a).

The British DI families were followed up when the children were aged 12 in order to assess the pattern of disclosure in these families, the main reasons for parents' decision to tell or not to tell their child about the way in which they were conceived, and whether or not parents' attitudes towards disclosure were any different now that their child was approaching adolescence (MacCallum et al., 2001; Golombok et al., 2002a). The results showed that only two (5.4 per cent) sets of parents had told their child about their donor origins and two other sets of parents stated that they were definitely planning to tell the child but had not yet done so. The large majority of the families (78.4 per cent) reported that they had definitely decided not to tell their child, and four (10.8 per cent) were still undecided. When asked to give the main reasons for their non-disclosure, the majority of parents (72 per cent) cited a desire to protect their child from the distress that may be caused by either finding out that their social father is not their genetic father or the inability to trace the donor because of the lack of available information. The belief that there was simply no need to tell the child was reported by 62 per cent of parents as another reason for their non-disclosure. Finally, almost half (46 per cent) of parents reported a desire to protect the father, which stemmed from the fear that the child would reject the father if he or she were to know the truth about his or her donor origins.

At the 12-year follow-up of the European DI families a strikingly similar pattern of findings emerged (Golombok et al., 2002b), only 8 (8.6 per cent) of the 102 DI families had told their child about the way in which they had been conceived (five in the Netherlands, two in the UK, one in Spain and none in Italy).

Parents' reasons for non-disclosure are surprisingly consistent across the different European samples, and their decision-making processes appear to involve the complex interaction of sociocultural factors (i.e. the stigma associated with male infertility), and more personal, familial factors (i.e. to protect the child and father–child relationship), a finding consistent with that reported elsewhere in the literature (Rowland, 1985; Nachtigall et al., 1997). In addition, parents' reasons for non-disclosure appear to be consistent over time, with the exception of uncertainty about the best time and method of telling children, which was important to parents when their child was aged between 4 and 8 years (Cook et al., 1995), but not by the time their child was aged 12 (MacCallum et al., 2001). Unlike adopted parents, DI parents lack the available scripts to guide them through the disclosure process and the use of an anonymous donor means that they have little information to give to the child about his or her genetic father. DI parents seem to experience more difficulties with disclosure (i.e. when and how to tell their child) when their child is young, but, by the time their child approaches adolescence, seem to have decided that non-disclosure is the best option for both the father and the child.

These findings are in line with those published elsewhere in the literature, which consistently show, even in the most recent studies, that despite increasing calls for sharing information with gamete donation children about the method of their conception, the majority of parents with a child conceived by DI still prefer to withhold such information from their child (Nachtigall, 1993; Klock et al., 1994; Brewaeys, 1996; Brewaeys et al., 1997a; Nachtigall et al., 1997). Indeed, in countries where children have the legal right to know the identity of the donor, such as Sweden, almost all parents continue to favour a position of non-disclosure to their child (Gottlieb et al., 2000).

Much less is known about the pattern of disclosure and the decision-making process of egg donation parents. To the extent that these families are similar to DI families with respect to the absence of a genetic link between one parent and the child, a similar pattern of disclosure may be expected among egg donation parents. However, other authors have argued that egg donation parents would be expected to be more open with their child on the grounds that egg donation is a more socially accepted procedure than DI (Haimes, 1993), and that the mothers' experience of pregnancy and childbirth would make the absence of a genetic relationship with their child less important (Greenfield et al., 1998).

To address these issues, the British group of 21 egg donation mothers of 3- to 8-year-old children were asked about whether or not they had told their child and other friends and family members, and their reasons for this decision (Golombok et al., 1999). It was found that only one set of egg donation parents had told their child, although 71 per cent of parents had told a friend or family member. When asked to elaborate on their reasons for this non-disclosure, the majority of parents (64 per cent) reported a wish to avoid distressing the child. Another 64 per cent of parents felt that there was no need to tell the child, which often stemmed from the mothers' experiences of carrying and giving birth to their child. The additional biological link with their children appeared to make it easier for egg donation mothers to 'forget' about the use of the donor egg (Murray and Golombok, 2001).

These findings contradict the conclusions drawn from previous research, which show that egg donation parents are more likely to disclose to their child information about their donor origins (Kirkland et al., 1992; Pettee and Weckstein, 1993; Weil et al., 1994; Greenfield et al., 1998). However, it must be pointed out that the higher levels of disclosure found in previous studies tended to be associated with the use of a known donor (usually a friend or relative). As the large majority of children in the present study were conceived using an egg from an anonymous donor, this suggests that these parents are more similar to DI parents in their decision not to tell.

Egg donation parents' reasons for non-disclosure when their children were aged between 3 and 8 years old were also similar to those of DI parents, with most parents concerned that disclosure would be detrimental to their child's happiness and psychological adjustment. They differed, however, in that egg donation parents were more likely to report at this stage that there was simply no need to tell the child, because of the mother's experience of carrying and giving birth to her child. As in DI families fathers lack such a biological link with their child, DI parents may give more thought to whether or not to disclose during the child's early years in contrast to egg donation parents for whom this appears to be less of an issue.

To the extent that similarities are drawn between gamete donation families and adopted families in terms of disclosure to the children, the findings suggest that gamete donation parents' reasons for non-disclosure are directly related to those areas in which DI and egg donation differ from adoption: acknowledgement of the father's infertility problem, the biological link between the mother and the child, the best time and way in which to tell the child, and the lack of information to give to the child about the donor (Cook et al., 1995; Murray and Golombok, 2001).

With respect to the psychological impact of non-disclosure on the children, findings from the European study suggest that non-disclosure does not appear to have a detrimental effect on children's social and emotional well-being; children aged between 4 and 8 do not experience raised levels of psychological problems and continue to function well at age 12 (Golombok et al., 1996, 1999, 2002a, 2002b). However, this does not necessarily mean that it is better not to inform children about their donor origins. It is important to remember that many parents had told other people, creating the possibility of the child finding out from another source. It is also plausible that the recent advances made in the field of genetic testing in medicine may place children at risk of finding out the truth about their donor origins later in life, and by someone other than their parents. Moreover, the consequences of non-disclosure in later adolescence and adulthood are not known.

As so few gamete donation children have been told about their genetic origins, it has not been possible systematically to assess the impact of disclosure versus non-disclosure on children's psychological adjustment. Evidence from the adoption literature provides useful guidelines for negotiating the disclosure process, suggesting that children are more likely to respond positively to such information if it is introduced early on in life and if parents continue to communicate openly with their child on this topic (Dudley and Neave, 1997). Anecdotal evidence shows that the same may also be true for gamete donation children, with some donor offspring who had found out in adulthood about the way in which they were conceived reporting feelings of hostility and distrust towards their parents (Cordray, 1999; Turner and Coyle, 2000), whereas those who had been told in childhood were generally accepting of this information (Snowden et al., 1983). Thus, greater difficulties might be expected for gamete donation children if they were to discover the truth about their donor origins later on in life.

Lesbian mother families

The 1970s saw the emergence of a new social phenomenon as an increasing number of lesbian women began fighting for the custody of their children when they divorced. At the time these women generally lost custody of their children on the basis that it would be detrimental for their child to be raised by a lesbian mother for two main reasons. First, it was argued that the children would be rejected by their peers and would suffer from psychological problems as a result. Second, it was assumed that children raised by a lesbian mother would show atypical sex development (i.e. that boys would be less masculine in their behaviour and identity and girls would be less feminine than children raised by heterosexual parents) and would be more likely to identify as gay or lesbian in adulthood, an outcome regarded as negative by the courts of law.

The impact of growing up in a lesbian family on children's sex development has been the topic of most debate in the discussion of lesbian mothers and their children. Within the literature sex development is generally thought to constitute three elements:

1. Sex identity (an individual's concept of him- or herself as male or female).
2. Sex role (those behaviours and attitudes considered appropriate to males and females within a given culture).
3. Sexual orientation (an individual's attraction to partners of the same sex [lesbian or gay] or the opposite sex [heterosexual]).

The degree to which being raised by a lesbian mother is thought to have an adverse effect on children's sex identity, sex role behaviour and sexual orientation varies according to the extent to which parents are thought to influence their child's sex development. One view, for example, is that sex development is biologically determined, influenced by different levels of prenatal sex hormones (e.g. testosterone) in the developing foetus (Collaer and Hines, 1995). In this case, parental behaviour and the family environment are assigned a minimal role in children's sex development.

The three most popular psychological theories of sex development (i.e. cognitive developmental, social learning and psychoanalytic theory) also differ in the extent to which parental factors are thought to play a role (see Golombok, 1999 for a review). According to traditional psychoanalytic theory, heterosexual parents are of central importance to children's sex development, particularly for ensuring the successful negotiation of the Oedipal phase, which culminates in girls' and boys' appropriate identification with the same sex parent, the adoption of male/female characteristics, and a heterosexual orientation later in life (Freud, 1905/1953, 1920/1955; Socarides, 1978). For children growing up in a lesbian family, psychoanalytic theorists would predict that the lack of a father figure means that boys would not identify with the male role and would be less masculine, and that girls, in identifying with a mother who has adopted a non-traditional female role, would be less feminine. Such a situation would also increase the likelihood of both boys and girls developing a homosexual orientation later in life (Socarides, 1978). Similarly, classic social learning theorists argue that heterosexual parents provide children with appropriate models for sex role behaviour and reinforce such behaviour in their children, and thus are a necessary prerequisite for their typical sex development (Mischel, 1970; Bandura, 1977).

More recently, contemporary social learning theorists have argued that other models and reinforcing agents, such as peers and sex stereotypes, are also important in children's acquisition of sex roles (Perry and Bussey, 1979; Bussey and Bandura, 1984; Bandura, 1986; Maccoby, 1992). In general, social learning theorists would expect children raised by lesbian mothers to experience different patterns of reinforcement than children from heterosexual families. Specifically, children in lesbian families may be less likely to be discouraged from exhibiting non-traditional sex role behaviour, or may have more flexible views of what constitutes male and female behaviour and be more accepting of behaviour that does not adhere to conventional sex stereotypes. Cognitive developmental theorists, on the other hand, assign parents a minimal role in children's sex development. According to this theory, children play an active role in obtaining and integrating information about gender from their wider social environment, and constructing for themselves what it means to be a boy or a girl (Stagnor and Ruble, 1987). From a cognitive developmental perspective, children from lesbian families would not be expected to be different from children from heterosexual families with regard to the process of integrating information from the wider environment and forming a view of themselves as male or female. Such conflicting views about parental influence on children's acquisition of sex roles means that it is not possible to make any clear predictions about the sex development of children raised in lesbian families.

As discussed earlier, parental responsiveness and emotional availability to the child are crucial for the development of secure attachment relationships and, ultimately, for children's psychological adjustment (Bowlby, 1969, 1988). Thus, children from lesbian families would not necessarily be expected to experience problems unless lesbian mothers differ from heterosexual mothers with regard to those aspects of parenting. However, it is important to note that children raised by lesbian mothers are more likely to have been exposed to known risk factors for childhood psychological disorder, such as parental divorce and single parenthood (McLanahan and Sandefur, 1994; Amato, 1993; Hetherington et al., 1998; Hetherington and Stanley-Hagan, 1999), although these risk factors are not related to lesbian mother families in and of themselves. The prediction that children growing up in lesbian families would be more at risk for behavioural and emotional problems is associated with the belief that they will be teased about their mother's sexual orientation and rejected by their peers. From a psychological perspective, it is generally acknowledged that satisfactory relationships with peers plays an important role in children's positive social and emotional development (Kupersmidt et al., 1990; Dunn and McGuire, 1992). Thus, difficulties would be expected for children growing up in a lesbian family to the extent that this experience interrupts the development of positive relationships with their peers.

The first studies of the development of children in lesbian mother families began in the 1970s and focused on those aspects of children's development that were the subject of most concern in child custody

cases: children's sex development and their overall psychological adjustment. Almost all of these early studies compared children raised by
lesbian mothers with children raised by a single heterosexual mother (see
Falk, 1989; Patterson, 1992; Golombok and Tasker, 1994 for reviews), the
reason being that the two types of family were the same in that the children were raised by women in the absence of a father, but were dissimilar
in terms of the sexual orientation of the mother. Employing this research
design allows the impact of the mothers' sexual orientation on children's
development to be assessed without the confounding effect of the presence of a father at home while the child is growing up. Findings from one
of the first systematic studies of single and lesbian mothers and their 10-
to 11-year-old children showed that none of the children exhibited any
sex identity confusion (i.e. none of the children expressed a desire to be
the other sex, or consistently exhibited cross-gender behaviour).
Furthermore, no differences were found between either boys or girls of
single heterosexual and lesbian mothers with regard to sex role.
Daughters of lesbian mothers were no less feminine and the sons were no
less masculine than their peers raised by heterosexual mothers
(Golombok et al., 1983).

Considering the children's general psychological adjustment, these
authors also reported that children from lesbian families were no more
likely to be teased or bullied by their peers than children from single
mother families, and children from both family types experienced good
quality friendships with their peers. Moreover, children raised by lesbian
mothers did not show a higher incidence of psychological disorder, as
rated blind by a child psychiatrist, than children raised by single heterosexual mothers (Golombok et al., 1983). Other studies have
demonstrated a similar pattern of findings regarding children's psychological well-being, irrespective of differences in the demographic
characteristics of the samples (Kirkpatrick et al., 1981; Green et al., 1986;
Huggins, 1989). Thus, it would appear that, for school-aged children,
being raised by a lesbian mother does not confer any particular risk for
atypical sex development or difficulties in peer relationships.

However, it is important to establish whether such positive outcomes
are found because these children pass through adolescence and into
adulthood or whether difficulties in psychological adjustment and intimate relationships arise as they grow up. Findings from a longitudinal
study of men and women who had grown up as children in lesbian families demonstrated that these young people continued to function well in
adulthood, experienced positive relationships with their mother and her
partner, and were no more likely to have been teased by peers in
adolescence (Tasker and Golombok, 1995, 1997). Although more of the

young people raised by lesbian mothers than heterosexual mothers had experimented with same-sex relationships, almost all of them identified as heterosexual in adulthood (Golombok and Tasker, 1996). Thus, being raised by a lesbian mother does not necessarily mean that children will identify as gay or lesbian themselves.

With regard to the quality of parenting in lesbian mother families, findings from a series of studies have consistently shown that lesbian mothers are just as warm and responsive to their children (Golombok et al., 1983), just as child centred (Miller et al., 1981; Kirkpatrick, 1987) and just as nurturing (Mucklow and Phelan, 1979) as their single heterosexual counterparts.

The increased availability of assisted reproductive techniques in the past 20 years has allowed a growing number of single lesbian women and lesbian couples access to DI in order to have a child, and a number of controlled studies of children raised in these types of family, compared with children raised in two-parent heterosexual families with a DI child, have recently been reported. Unlike children in the early studies of lesbian families, DI children born to lesbian mothers are raised from birth without a father in the family home, so it is possible to assess directly the impact of the mother's sexual orientation on their psychological development. In a British study (Golombok et al., 1997) of 30 lesbian mother families and 41 two-parent heterosexual families, we assessed the quality of parenting and the social and emotional development of the child using a combination of standardized interview and questionnaire measures. Similar studies have also been carried out in Belgium (Brewaeys et al., 1997a, 1997b) and the USA (Flaks et al., 1995; Chan et al., 1998).

Taken together, the findings from these studies suggest that children raised by lesbian mothers from birth are no different in terms of their sex identity and sex role behaviour than their peers from two-parent heterosexual families. Thus, the presence of a father does not appear to be a necessary prerequisite for the children's development of sex-typed behaviour, nor does a mother's lesbian sexual orientation in itself appear to interfere with her children's sex development. All these children, however, had some contact with men and, in many cases, experienced a close relationship with at least one of the mothers' male friends. Regarding general psychological adjustment, all of the children appeared to be functioning well, with no greater incidence of behavioural or emotional problems among children raised from birth by lesbian mothers. This may result, in part, from the fact that almost all these children were raised in an intact two-parent family, where a good relationship existed between the parents, and the children had not been exposed to the potentially negative effects associated with parental divorce and separation, a common experience of children in studies of other fatherless families (Golombok, 1999). However, all the children studied to date are still relatively young (i.e. school-age), and it remains to be seen whether this positive pattern of results prevails as the children make the transition through adolescence and into young adulthood.

The issue of disclosure about the use of donated sperm is also relevant to lesbian families; like heterosexual DI parents, lesbian DI mothers must decide whether or not they are going to inform their child about their donor origins. As previously noted, the majority of heterosexual DI parents choose not to tell their child about the way in which they were conceived (Brewaeys, 1996; Nachtigall, 1993; Klock et al., 1994; Brewaeys et al., 1997a/b; Nachtigall et al., 1997), attributing their non-disclosure to factors such as a wish to avoid distressing their child, to protect the relationship between the non-genetic father and the child, and to protect the father from the negative stigma of male infertility (Cook et al., 1995; MacCallum et al., 2001). It has been suggested that the lack of a father figure in lesbian families means that lesbian mothers would be more likely to inform their child about the use of donated sperm.

Findings from a number of studies employing samples from different countries, such as Belgium and Canada, have consistently confirmed this view; almost all lesbian DI mothers, in contrast to heterosexual DI parents, have told or plan to tell their child about their donor origins. Among those mothers who had already told, disclosure most often occurred in early childhood, within the context of explaining to the child about their family structure (i.e. the absence of a father) and was related to the intention to be open with their child about their sexual orientation (Brewaeys et al., 1993, 1997a/b; Dundas and Kaufman, 2000; Vanfraussen et al., 2001).

Interestingly, the high levels of disclosure in lesbian DI families did not appear to be related to a greater desire to use an identifiable donor. In most cases, lesbian mothers preferred to use an anonymous donor in order to avoid any interference in the family by a third party, a situation that most mothers thought would be detrimental to their child's psychological well-being (Brewaeys et al., 1993; Dundas and Kaufman, 2000). However, findings from later research suggest that mothers' views on the identity of the donor may change over time. For example one follow-up study of 50 lesbian DI families in Belgium showed that at the time of insemination only 10 per cent of parents were in favour of registration of the identity of the donor. By the time their child was aged between 1 and 2 years, this figure had significantly increased to 56 per cent, suggesting that once the child was born parents were more likely to consider the child's point of view (i.e. anticipating that the child might want information about the donor) (Brewaeys et al., 1995).

The trend towards disclosure in lesbian DI families provides a unique opportunity to assess the impact of knowledge about their donor origins on children's psychological well-being, as well as mothers' and children's views of the donor. As discussed above, DI children raised by lesbian mothers appear to be functioning well, suggesting that these school-age children are not experiencing any difficulties in coming to terms with information about their donor origins. However, whether or not lesbian mothers continue to employ an open, non-defensive communication style when discussing the donor with their children as they grow up, a factor that has been shown to be associated with healthy identity development in adopted children (Brodzinsky et al., 1995), remains to be established.

With respect to the mothers' and children's views of the donor, one recent study by Vanfraussen et al. (2001) of 45 lesbian parents and 41 children aged between 7 and 17 years in Belgium found that, within families, mothers' and children's concepts of the donor may differ. Although the majority of mothers had explained the use of a donor as 'buying or getting some seeds', thereby reducing the donor to an anonymous sperm cell, nearly half the children expressed an interest in finding out about the 'man' or 'unknown father' who had donated his sperm. However, they varied in the type of information they wanted to be made available to them. This ranged from non-identifying characteristics, such as the donor's physical appearance and personality traits, to the actual identity of the donor. Of those children who were curious to know the identity of the donor, more boys than girls wanted this information, which may be the result of the absence of a father in lesbian families. Thus, family structure may influence DI children's views of the amount and type of information about the donor that they would want to be made available to them. A different pattern of results might be expected in father-present families.

Based on the collective evidence above, disclosure about DI in lesbian families does not appear to affect the children negatively. However, the nature of the relationship of children's response to knowledge about the donor, their view of the donor, and measures of their social and emotional development remain to be directly assessed. Furthermore, as hereditary links are thought to form the basis of one's view of the self and identity (Cohen, 1996), it is important to establish whether the absence of identifying information about the donor will have an adverse effect on children's psychological well-being. None of the children studied had reached adulthood and it is possible that the genetic link with the donor may become more important to them as they mature or when, as adults, they consider having children of their own and issues of heredity and paternity become more salient.

Single mother families

It is estimated that in the UK approximately 22 per cent of families, and roughly one-quarter of families in the USA, are headed by a single mother (ONS, 2002; Burns, 1992; Roll, 1992). Although most of these families occur as a direct result of parental divorce or separation, an increasing number of single heterosexual women are choosing to become mothers without living with the father of their child (Burghes, 1993), or are visiting infertility clinics and requesting DI so that they may have a child without any involvement of a male partner (Shenfield, 1994). As a result, there are a growing number of children who are being raised by 'solo mothers', i.e. mothers who are choosing to rear their child from birth without a male partner.

The first studies of the impact of growing up without a father on children's psychological well-being focused almost exclusively on those children who had lived with both their mother and their father early on in life and then, after experiencing a parental divorce or separation, grew up living only with their mother. Findings from this early research demonstrated that the absence of a father had a detrimental effect on children's cognitive and socioemotional development (see Herzog and Sudia, 1973; Biller, 1974 for a review). Later research suggests that the relationship between these factors may, in fact, be more complex, e.g. one common consequence of single parenthood, particularly after the separation/divorce of two parents, is financial hardship and lower social class. A number of investigators have found that, after controlling for these social/economic factors, the absence of a father does not exert any negative effect on children's intellectual ability or social adjustment (Broman et al., 1975; Ferri, 1976; Crockett et al., 1993). Drawing on findings from a number of representative American samples of single mother families, McLanahan and Sandefur (1994) further suggested that the lower income associated with single parenthood is the most influential factor in the later underachievement of children raised in these families. Another consequence of single parenthood is lack of social support, which has been shown to be associated with difficulties in parenting for some single mothers (Weinraub and Gringlas, 1995). Thus, it would appear that social/economic disadvantages related to single parenthood are more likely to have a negative impact on children's psychological well-being and quality of parenting than the absence of a father as such.

Other factors thought to contribute to the negative outcomes for children raised by single mothers are associated with the reasons for becoming a single parent family, such as death of a parent or divorce, and the length of time preceding the transition from a two-parent to a fatherless family. Studies comparing the effect of parental divorce with the death of a father on children's psychological development have found that those children who had experienced a divorce or separation were more likely to exhibit behavioural problems and to experience difficulties in the transition from adolescence to adulthood (Rutter, 1971; Ferri, 1976; McLanahan and Sandefur, 1994). After reviewing the research of the effects of parental divorce on children's psychological adjustment, Amato (1993) concluded that it is conflict between parents that is the most likely cause of emotional distress among children of divorce. In addition, evidence from longitudinal studies of divorced and intact families conducted in the UK and the USA shows that the presence of children's behavioural problems and general difficulties in family functioning before the parents' separation or divorce were strongly related to children's difficulties in the aftermath of the family break-up (Cherlin et al., 1991). Thus, factors that predate, rather than occur as a result of, the fatherless family may also play an important role in children's later psychological adjustment.

Although there is much research on children raised by single heterosexual mothers who had lived with their father during their first years of life, very few studies have assessed children raised by 'solo' mothers (i.e. mothers who raise their child from birth without a male partner), including mothers who have undergone DI in order to have a child. As children raised by solo mothers will not have experienced a parental divorce or separation, which, in itself, might render children vulnerable to the development of psychological problems (Amato and Keith, 1991), the findings from existing research cannot be generalized to this group of families.

Children raised from birth without a father may not be any more at risk for social and emotional problems than children from intact two-parent heterosexual families as neither group will have endured parental conflict and the break-up of the family. However, solo mothers may be more vulnerable to other factors, such as social stigma and lack of social support, which might adversely affect their parenting ability, leading to social and emotional problems for their children (Golombok, 1999). Findings from one British general population study of children raised from birth by a single heterosexual mother tentatively suggested that these children were functioning just as well as children in two-parent families (Ferri, 1976). Other studies have shown more negative outcomes for children of solo mothers, but these seem to be related to the social and economic factors cited above, such as financial hardship and lack of social support, rather than the absence of a father in itself (McLananhan and Sandefur, 1994; Weinraub and Gringlas, 1995). Such evidence has helped fuel a negative social stereotype of single mothers, particularly those who are financially dependent on the state, as being responsible for creating an 'underclass' of drug addicts and delinquents. However, in a study of middle-class mothers who were financially secure and who had raised their child alone from the first year of their child's life, we found these children to be more securely attached to their mothers, and no more likely to show psychological problems than a matched group of children from two-parent families (Golombok et al., 1997a/b). It is important to bear in mind that the social and economic circumstances of single mothers and the outcomes for children may be as varied as those of two-parent families. Future research must attempt to identify those factors associated with single parenthood that may render children vulnerable to psychological problems and those that do not place the child at risk.

Although there is a growing number of single heterosexual women undergoing DI in order to have a child, the issue of whether this group of women should be given access to such assisted reproductive techniques remains a topic of much debate (Englert, 1994; Shenfield, 1994). Findings from a small sample of 10 single women requesting DI showed that a common reason for choosing this method of conception was to avoid either having a man's child without his knowledge or consent, or having to share the responsibilities for the child with a man with whom they were not having a relationship (cited by Fidell and Marik, 1989) To date, no studies exist of children raised by single mothers who have used some form of assisted reproductive technique in order to conceive their child. These children will not have experienced a parental divorce and the ensuing disruption in family relationships, reducing the potentially negative consequences for these children. Moreover, anecdotal evidence suggests that solo mother DI families are generally financially secure, which may be result partly from the forethought involved when single women actively choose to conceive and raise a child on their own. On the other hand, little is known about the potential effect of negative social stigma and the absence of a second parent to share the load. The impact on the child's psychological development of disclosure or non-disclosure about the child's origins are also relevant to solo mother children conceived by DI. To address these issues, we are currently conducting a study of solo mothers and their DI children at City University, London.

Conclusions

The emergence of new types of families – assisted reproduction families, planned lesbian mother families and single mother families – have raised a number of concerns about potentially negative implications for parenting and children's psychological development, e.g. it has been argued that the absence of a father in lesbian and solo mother families may have a detrimental effect on children's psychological well-being, and families created by assisted reproduction may be characterized by dysfunctional parenting related to parents' inability to come to terms with their infertility and the stress associated with infertility treatment. In the case of gamete donation families, it has been argued that a missing genetic link between the parent and the child may cause problems in the relationship between the non-genetic parent and the child. Based on existing evidence, however, it would seem that these concerns have not materialized. Parents and children in these new types of family appear to experience warm, loving relationships and the children show no evidence of psychological problems. The findings suggest that a positive family environment is more important for children's psychological well-being than their family structure, i.e. whether they have one parent or two, whether their parents are heterosexual or homosexual, and whether or not they are genetically related to one or both of their parents (Golombok, 2000).

Nevertheless, it must be borne in mind that this is a relatively new field of research and, as a result, few systematic, controlled studies have assessed the outcomes for these families as the children pass through adolescence and into adulthood. Thus, much remains to be determined about how these children fare as adults. Specifically, to what extent, and how, will their family experiences affect their own parenting behaviour? Will their attitudes about growing up in a particular type of family change when they become parents themselves? What will happen if they find out as adults that one or both of their parents is not genetically related to them? Moreover, consideration of the effects of the specific sociocultural context in which these families are created and exist is also important. More accepting cultural attitudes towards assisted reproduction are likely to have a positive effect on family life.

References

Achilles R (1992) Donor Insemination: An overview. Royal Commission on New Reproductive Technologies. Ontario, Canada.

Amato P (1993) Children's adjustment to divorce: Theories, hypotheses, and empirical support. Journal of Marriage and the Family 55: 23–38.

Amato PR, Keith B (1991) Parental divorce and the well-being of children: A meta-analysis. Psychological Bulletin 110: 26–46.

Bandura A (1977) Social Learning Theory. Englewood Cliffs, NJ: Prentice Hall.

Bandura A (1986) Social Foundations of Thought and Action: A social cognitive theory. Englewood Cliffs, NJ: Prentice Hall.

Baran A, Pannor R (1993) Lethal Secrets. New York: Amistad.

Baumrind D (1989) Rearing competent children. In Damon W (ed.), Child Development Today and Tomorrow. San Francisco: Jossey-Bass, pp. 349–378.

Biller HB (1974) Parental Deprivation. Lexington, Mass: Heath.

Bok S (1982) Secrets. New York: Pantheon.

Bowlby J (1969) Attachment and Loss, Vol. 1. Attachment. London: Hogarth Press.

Bowlby J (1973) Attachment and Loss, Vol. 2. Separation. London: Hogarth Press.

Bowlby J (1988) A Secure Base: Clinical applications of attachment theory. London: Routledge.

Brandes JM, Scher A, Itzkovits J, Thaler I, Sarid M, Gershoni-Baruch R (1992) Growth and development of children conceived by in vitro fertilization. Pediatrics 90: 424–429.

Brewaeys A (1996) Donor insemination, the impact on family and child development. Journal of Psychosomatic Obstetrics and Gynecology 17: 1–13.

Brewaeys A, Ponjaert-Kristoffersen I, Van Steirteghem, Devroey P (1993) Children from anonymous donors: an inquiry into homosexual and heterosexual parents' attitudes. Journal of Psychosomatic Obstetrics and Gynecology 14: 23–35.

Brewaeys A, Devroey P, Helmerhorst FM, Van Hall EV, Ponjaert I (1995) Lesbian mothers who conceived after donor insemination: a follow-up study. Human Reproduction 10: 2731–2725.

Brewaeys A, Golombok S, Naaktgeboren N, de Bruyn JK, Van Hall EV (1997a) Donor insemination: Dutch parents' opinions about confidentiality and donor anonymity and the emotional adjustment of their children. Human Reproduction 12: 1591–1597.

Brewaeys A, Ponjaert-Kristoffersen I, Van Hall EV, Golombok S (1997b) Donor insemination: Child development and family functioning in lesbian mother families. Human Reproduction 12: 1349–1359.

Brodzinsky DM, Lang R, Smith DW (1995) Parenting adopted children. In: Bornstein M (ed.), Handbook of Parenting. Hove: Lawrence Erlbaum Associates, pp. 209–232.

Broman SH, Nichols PL, Kennedy WA (1975) Pre-School IQ: Parental and early development correlates. Hillsdale, NJ: Erlbaum.

Burghes L (1993) One-parent Families: Policy options for the 1990's. York: Joseph Rowntree Foundation/Maxiprint.

Burns A (1992) Mother-headed families: an international perspective and the case of Australia. Social Policy Report 4(1): 1–24.

Burns LH (1990) An exploratory study of perceptions of parenting after infertility. Family Systems Medicine 8(2): 177–189.

Bussey K, Bandura A (1984) Influence of gender constancy and social power on sex-linked modeling. Journal of Personality and Social Psychology 47: 1292–1302.

Cederblad M, Friberg B, Ploman F, Sjoberg NO, Stjernqvist K, Zackrisson E (1996) Intelligence and behaviour in children born after in-vitro fertilization treatment. Human Reproduction 11: 2052–2057.

Chan RW, Raboy B, Patterson CJ (1998) Psychosocial adjustment among children conceived via donor insemination by lesbian and heterosexual mothers. Child Development 69: 443–457.

Cherlin A, Furstenberg F, Chase-Lansdale P et al. (1991) Longitudinal studies of effects of divorce on children in Great Britain and the United States. Science 252: 1386–1389.

Clamar A (1989) Psychological implications of the anonymous pregnancy. In: Offerman-Zuckerberg J (ed.), Gender in Transition: A new frontier. New York: Plenum Medical Book Co.

Cohen BC (1996) Parents anonymous. New ways of making babies. In: Cohen BC (ed.), The Case of Egg Donation. Indiana: Indiana University Press, pp. 88–105.

Collaer ML, Hines M (1995) Human behavioural sex differences: A role for gender hormones during early development? Psychological Bulletin 118: 55–107.

Colpin H, Demyttenaere K, Vandemeulebroecke L (1995) New reproductive technology and the family: the parent–child relationship following *in vitro* fertilization. Journal of Child Psychology and Psychiatry 36: 1429–1441.

Cook R, Golombok S, Bish A, Murray C (1995) Keeping Secrets: A controlled study of parental attitudes towards telling in donor insemination families. American Journal of Orthopsychiatry 65: 549–559.

Cook R, Parsons J, Mason B, Golombok S (1989) Emotional, marital and sexual functioning in patients embarking on IVF and AID treatment for infertility. Journal of Reproductive and Infant Psychology 7: 87–93.

Cordray B (1999) Speaking for ourselves: Quotes from men and women created by DI/remote father conception. 11th World Congress on In Vitro Fertilization and Human Reproductive Genetics, Sydney, Australia.

Cox MJ, Owen MT, Lewis JM, Henderson VK (1989) Marriage, adult adjustment, and early parenting. Child Development 60: 1015–1024.

Crockett LJ, Eggebeen DJ, Hawkins AJ (1993) Fathers' presence and young children's behavioral and cognitive adjustment. Journal of Family Issues 14: 355–377.

Daniels KR (1995) Information sharing in donor insemination: A conflict of rights and needs. Cambridge Quarterly of Healthcare Ethics 4: 217–224.

Daniels KR, Taylor K (1993) Secrecy and openness in donor insemination. Politics and Life Sciences 12: 155–170.

Dudley M, Neave G (1997) Issues for families and children where conception was achieved using donor gametes. In: Lorbach C (ed.), Let the Offspring Speak: Discussions on Donor Conception. Australia: Donor Conception Support Group of Australia, pp. 125–126.

Dundas S, Kaufman M (2000) The Toronto Lesbian Family Study. Journal of Homosexuality 40(2): 65–79.

Dunn J, McGuire S (1992) Sibling and peer relationships in childhood. Journal of Child Psychology and Psychiatry 33: 67–105.

Dyer C (2000) Offspring from artificial insemination demand father's details. British Medical Journal 312: 654.

Englert Y (1994) Artificial insemination of single women and lesbian women with donor sperm. Human Reproduction 9: 1969–1971.

Falk PJ (1989) Lesbian mothers, psychosocial assumptions in family law. American Psychologist 44: 941–947.

Ferri E (1976) Growing Up in a One Parent Family. Slough: National Foundation for Educational Research.

Fidell L, Marik J (1989) Paternity by proxy: artificial insemination by donor sperm. In: Offerman-Zuckerbery J (ed.), Gender in Transition: A new frontier. New York: Plenum.

Flaks DK, Ficher I, Masterpasqua F, Joseph G (1995) Lesbians choosing motherhood: a comparative study of lesbian and heterosexual parents and their children. Developmental Psychology 31: 105–114.

Freud S (1905/1953) Three Essays on the Theory of Sexuality. London: Hogarth Press.

Freud S (1920/1955) Beyond the Pleasure Principle. London: Hogarth Press.

Gibson FL, Ungerer JA, Leslie GI, Saunders DM, Tennant CC (1998) Development, behaviour and temperament: a prospective study of infants conceived through in-vitro fertilization. Human Reproduction 13: 1727–1732.

Golombok S (1999) New family forms: children raised in solo mother families, lesbian mother families, and in families created by assisted reproduction. In: Balter L, Tamis-LeMonda L (eds), Child Psychology: A handbook of contemporary issues. Philadelphia, Pa: Psychology Press, pp. 429–446.

Golombok S (2000) Parenting: What really counts? London: Routledge.

Golombok S, Tasker F (1994) Children in lesbian and gay families: theories and evidence. Annual Review of Sex Research 4: 73–100.

Golombok S, Tasker F (1996) Do parents influence the sexual orientation of their children? Findings from a longitudinal study of lesbian families. Developmental Psychology 32: 3–11.

Golombok S, Spencer A, Rutter M (1983) Children in lesbian and single-parent households: psychosexual and psychiatric appraisal. Journal of Child Psychology and Psychiatry 24: 551–572.

Golombok S, Cook R, Bish A, Murray C (1995) Families created by the new reproductive technologies: quality of parenting and social and emotional development of the children. Child Development 66: 285–298.

Golombok S, Brewaeys A, Cook R et al. (1996) The European Study of Assisted Reproduction Families: family functioning and child development. Human Reproduction 11: 101.

Golombok S, Tasker F, Murray C (1997) Children raised in fatherless families from infancy: family relationships and the socioemotional development of children of lesbian and single heterosexual mothers. Journal of Child Psychology and Psychiatry 38: 783–792.

Golombok S, Murray C, Brinsden P, Abdalla H (1999) Social versus biological parenting: family functioning and the socioemotional development of children conceived by egg or sperm donation. Journal of Child Psychology and Psychiatry 40: 519–527.

Golombok S, MacCallum F, Goodman E (2001) The 'test-tube' generation: parent-child relationships and the psychological well-being of IVF children at adolescence. Child Development 72: 599–608

Golombok S, MacCallum F, Goodman E, Rutter M (2002a) Families with children conceived by donor insemination: a follow-up at age 12. Child Development 73: in press.

Golombok S, Brewaeys MT, Giavazzi D, Guerra D, MacCallum F, Rust J (2002b) The European Study of Assisted Reproduction Families: the transition to adolescence. Human Reproduction 17: 830–840.

Gottlieb C, Lalos O, Lindblad F (2000) Disclosure of donor insemination to the child: the impact of Swedish legislation on couples' attitudes. Human Reproduction 15: 2052–2056.

Green R, Mandel JB, Hotvedt ME, Gray J, Smith L (1986) Lesbian mothers and their children: a comparison with solo parent heterosexual mothers and their children. Archives of Sexual Behavior 15: 167–184.

Greenfield DA, Greenfield DG, Mazure CM, Keefe DL, Olive DL (1998) Do attitudes towards disclosure in donor oocyte recipients predict the use of anonymous versus directed donation? Fertility and Sterility 70: 1009–1014.

Grossmann KE, Grossmann K, Spangler G, Suess G, Unzler L (1985) Maternal sensitivity in northern Germany. Growing points of attachment theory and research. In: Bretherton I, Waters E (eds), Monographs of the Society for Research in Child Development, Vol. 50: (1–2, Serial No 209) 233–256.

Haimes E (1993) Do clinicians benefit from gamete donor anonymity? Human Reproduction 9: 1518–1520.

Herzog E, Sudia CE (1973) Children in fatherless families. In: Campbell BM, Riccuiti HN (eds), Review of Child Development Research. Chicago: University of Chicago Press.

Hetherington EM, Stanley-Hagan M (1999) The adjustment of children with divorced parents: a risk and resiliency perspective. Journal of Child Psychology and Psychiatry 40: 129–140.

Hetherington EM, Bridges M, Isabella GM (1998) What matters? What does not? Five perspectives on the association between marital transitions and children's adjustment. American Psychologist 53: 167–184.

Hoopes JL (1990) Adoption and identity formation. In: Brodzinsky DMS (ed.), The Psychology of Adoption. Oxford: Oxford University Press.

Howes P, Markman HJ (1989) Marital quality and child functioning: a longitudinal investigation. Child Development 60: 1044–1051.

Huggins SL (1989) A comparative study of self-esteem of adolescent children of divorced lesbian mothers and divorced heterosexual mothers. In: Bozett F (ed.), Homosexuality and the Family. New York: Harrington Park.

Kirkland A, Power M, Burton G, Baber R, Studd J, Abdalla H (1992) Comparison of attitudes of donors and recipients to oocyte donation. Human Reproduction 7: 355–357.

Kirkpatrick M (1987) Clinical implications of lesbian mother studies. Journal of Homosexuality 13: 201–211.

Kirkpatrick M, Smith C, Roy R (1981) Lesbian mothers and their children: a comparative survey. American Journal of Orthopsychiatry 51: 545–551.

Klock SC (1993) Psychological aspects of donor insemination. Infertility and Reproduction Clinics of North America 4: 455–469.

Klock SC, Jacob MC, Maier D (1994) A prospective study of donor insemination recipients: secrecy, privacy, and disclosure. Fertility and Sterility 62: 477–484.

Kovacs GT, Mushin D, Kane H, Baker HWG (1993) A controlled study of the psycho-social development of children conceived following insemination with donor semen. Human Reproduction 8: 788–790.

Kupersmidt JB, Coie JD, Dodge KA (1990) The role of poor peer relationships in the development of disorder. In: Asher SR, Coie JD (eds), Peer Rejection in Childhood. Cambridge: Cambridge University Press, pp. 274–305.

Landau R (1998) Secrecy, anonymity, and deception in donor insemination: a genetic, psycho-social and ethical critique. Social Work and Healthcare 28(1): 75–89.

Levy-Shiff R, Vakil E, Dimitrovsky L et al. (1998) Medical, cognitive, emotional, and behavioural outcomes in school-age children conceived by in-vitro fertilization. Journal of Clinical Child Psychology 27: 320–329.

Lutjen P, Trounson A, Leeton J, Findlay J, Wood C, Renou P (1984) The establishment and maintenance of pregnancy using in vitro fertilization and embryo donation in a patient with primary ovarian failure. Nature 307: 174–175.

MacCallum F, Goodman E, Kerai V, Golombok S (2001) Parents' attitudes towards disclosure in DI families. Paper presented at the 57th Annual meeting of the American Society of Reproductive Medicine, Florida, 20–25 October.

Maccoby EE (1992) The role of parents in the socialization of children. Developmental Psychology 28: 1006–1017.

McLanahan S, Sandefur G (1994) Growing Up with a Single Parent: What hurts, What helps. Cambridge, Mass: Harvard University Press.

McMahon C, Ungerer J, Beaurepaire J, Tennant C, Saunders D (1995) Psychosocial outcomes for parents and children after in vitro fertilization: a review. Journal of Reproductive and Infant Psychology 13: 1–16.

McMahon CA, Ungerer JA, Tennant C, Saunders D (1997) Psychosocial adjustment and the quality of the mother–child relationship at four months postpartum after conception by in vitro fertilization. Fertility and Sterility 68: 492–500.

Mahlstedt PP, Greenfield DA (1989) Assisted reproductive technology with donor gametes: the need for patient preparation. Fertility and Sterility 52: 908–914.

Main M, Kaplan N, Cassidy J (1985) Security in infancy, childhood and adulthood: a move to the level of representation. In: Bretherton I, Waters E (eds), Monographs of the Society for Research in Child Development 50: 66–104.

Maughan B, Pickles A (1990) Adopted and illegitimate children growing up. In: Robins LN, Rutter M (eds), Straight and Devious Pathways from Childhood to Adulthood. Cambridge: Cambridge University Press, pp. 36–61.

Miller BC, Fan X, Christensen M, Grotevant HD, van Dulmen M (2000) Comparisons of adopted and nonadopted adolescents in a large, nationally representative sample. Child Development 71: 1458–1473.

Miller JA, Jacobson RB, Bigner JJ (1981) The child's home environment for lesbian vs. heterosexual mothers: a neglected area of research. Journal of Homosexuality 7: 49–56.

Mischel W (1970) Sex-typing and socialization. In: Mussen P (ed.), Carmichael's Manual of Child Psychology, Vol. 2. New York: Wiley, pp. 3–72.

Morin NC, Wirth FH, Johnson DH et al. (1989) Congenital malformations and psychosocial development in children conceived by in vitro fertilization. Journal of Pediatrics 115: 222–227.

Mucklow BM, Phelan GK (1979) Lesbian and traditional mothers' responses to child behaviour and self-concept. Psychological Reports 44: 880–882.

Murray C, Golombok S (2001) To tell or not to tell: the decision-making process of egg donation parents. Paper presented at the 57th Annual meeting of the American Society of Reproductive Medicine, Florida, 20–25 October.

Mushin DN, Barreda-Hanson MC, Spensley JC (1986) In vitro fertilization children: early psychosocial development. Journal of In Vitro Fertilization and Embryo Transfer 3: 247–252.

Nachtigall RD (1993) Secrecy: an unresolved issue in donor insemination. American Journal of Obstetrics and Gynecology 169: 1846–1849.

Nachtigall RD, Becker G, Quiroga SS, Tschann JM (1997) The disclosure decision: concerns and issues of parents of children conceived through donor insemination. American Journal of Obstetrics and Gynecology 178: 1165–70.

Office of National Statistics (2002) Social Trends 32. HMSO, UK.

Olivennes F, Kerbrat V, Rufat P, Blanchet V, Franchin R, Frydman R (1997) Follow-up of a cohort of 422 children aged 6–13 years conceived by in vitro fertilization. Fertility and Sterility 67: 284–289.

Papaligouras Z (1998) The effects of in-vitro fertilization on parent–infant communication. Unpublished PhD thesis, University of Edinburgh.

Papp P (1993) The worm in the bud: secrets between parents and children. In: Imber-Black E (ed.), Secrets in Families and Family Therapy. New York: Norton, pp. 66–85.

Patterson CJ (1992) Children of lesbian and gay parents. Child Development 63: 1025–1042.

Perry DG, Bussey K (1979) The social learning theory of sex difference: imitation is alive and well. Journal of Personality and Social Psychology 37: 1699–1712.

Pettee D, Weckstein LN (1993) A survey of parental attitudes toward oocyte donation. Human Reproduction 8: 1963–1965.

Quinton D, Rutter M (1988) Parenting Breakdown: The making and breaking of intergenerational links. Aldershot: Avebury Gower Publishing.

Raoul-Duval A, Bertrand-Servais M, Frydman R (1993) Comparative prospective study of the psychological development of children born by in vitro fertilization and their mothers. Journal of Psychosomatic Obstetrics and Gynecology 14: 117–126.

Roll J (1992) Lone Parent Families in the European Community. London: European Family and Social Policy Unit.

Ron-El R, Lahat E, Golan A, Lerman M, Bukovsky I, Herman A (1994) Development of children born after ovarian superovulation induced by long-acting gonadatrophin-releasing hormone antagonists and menotrophins, and by in vitro fertilization. Journal of Pediatrics 125: 734–737.

Rowland R (1985) The social and psychological consequences of secrecy in AI by donor programmes. Social Science and Medicine 4: 391–396.

Rutter M (1971) Parent–child separation: psychological effects on children. Journal of Child Psychology and Psychiatry 12: 233–260.

Schechter MD, Bertocci D (1990) The meaning of the search. In: Brodzinshy DMS (ed.), The Psychology of Adoption. Oxford: Oxford University Press.

Shenfield F (1994) Filiation in assisted reproduction: potential conflicts and legal implications. Human Reproduction 9: 1348–1354.

Shenfield F, Steele SJ (1997) What are the effects of anonymity and secrecy on the welfare of the child in gamete donation? Human Reproduction 12: 392–395.

Singer L, Brodzinsky D, Ramsay D, Steir M, Waters E (1985) Mother–infant attachment in adoptive families. Child Development 56: 1543–1551.

Snowden R (1990) The family and artificial reproduction. In: Bromhan EA (ed.), Philosophical Ethics in Reproductive Medicine. Manchester: Manchester University Press.

Snowden R, Mitchell GD, Snowden EM (1983) Artificial Reproduction: A social investigation. London: George Allen & Unwin.

Socarides CW (1978) Homosexuality. New York: Jason Aronson.

Soderstrom-Antilla V, Sajaniemi N, Tiitinen A, Hovatta O (1998) Health and development of children born after oocyte donation compared with that of those born after in-vitro fertilization, and parents' attitudes regarding secrecy. Human Reproduction 13: 2009–2015.

Stagnor C, Ruble DM (1987) Development of gender role knowledge and gender constancy. In: Signorella LSLML (ed.), Children's Gender Schemata: New direction for child development. San Francisco: Jossey-Bass.

Steptoe PC, Edwards RG (1978) Birth after reimplantation of a human embryo. Lancet ii: 366.

Tasker F, Golombok S (1995) Adults raised as children in lesbian families. American Journal of Orthopsychiatry 65: 203–215.

Tasker F, Golombok S (1997) Growing up in a Lesbian Family. New York: Guilford Press.

Triseliotis J (1973) In Search of Origins: The experiences of adopted people. London: Routledge & Kegan Paul.

Turner AJ, Coyle A (2000) What does it mean to be a donor offspring? The identity experiences of adults conceived by donor insemination and the implications for counselling and therapy. Human Reproduction 15: 2041–2051.

van Balen F (1996) Child-rearing following in vitro fertilization. Journal of Child Psychology and Psychiatry 37: 687–693.

van Balen F (1998) Development of IVF children. Developmental Review 18: 30–46.

Vanfraussen K, Ponjaert-Kristoffersen I, Brewaeys A (2001) An attempt to reconstruct children's donor concept: a comparison between children's and lesbian parents' attitudes towards donor anonymity. Human Reproduction 16: 2019–2025.

Walker I, Broderick P (1999) The psychology of assisted reproduction – or psychology assisting its reproduction. Australian Psychologist 34(1): 38–44.

Weaver SM, Clifford E, Gordon AG, Hay DM, Robinson J (1993) A follow-up study of 'successful' IVF/GIFT couples: social-emotional well-being and adjustment to parenthood. Journal of Psychosomatic Obstetrics and Gynecology 14: 5–16.

Weil E, Cornet D, Sibony C, Mandelbaum J, Salat-Baroux J (1994) Psychological aspects in anonymous and non-anonymous oocyte donation. Human Reproduction 9: 1344–1347.

Weinraub M, Gringlas MB (1995) Single parenthood. In: Bornstein M (ed.), Handbook of Parenting. Hove: Lawrence Erlbaum Associates.

Yovich J, Parry T, French N, Grauaug A (1986) Developmental assessment of 20 in vitro fertilization (I.V.F.) infants at their first birthday. Journal of In Vitro Fertilization and Embryo Transfer 3: 225–237.

CHAPTER 7

Disclosure and development: 'taking the baby home was just the beginning'

ALEXINA M MCWHINNIE

The early debate in the 1970s and 1980s about the use of medical intervention to alleviate infertility and childlessness questioned the morality and ethics of the practice that had produced the first test-tube baby in 1978. Was it appropriate to produce and manipulate human embryos? There was deep concern about the children created in this way, and about the moral status of the embryo, and whether to prohibit, allow or regulate the practice of IVF (*in vitro* fertilization) and the development of third-party conception (i.e. the use of donor gametes). Since the political decision in the UK was to allow the practice but to regulate it through the Human Fertilisation and Embryology Act 1990, assisted human reproduction has expanded rapidly both in the public sector in the National Health Service and in the private fee-paying sector. The expressed doubts about its general use have faded under the pressure of a general and media consensus. Those who continue to oppose it find themselves in a minority and frequently linked to the anti-abortion lobby. Inevitably the two are associated, given their views on the sanctity of human life, but they are wrongly assumed to be the same. Such views that question current procedures and assumptions should be listened to and respected, because the psychological and ethical dilemmas have not gone away simply because it is now legal to continue the practice. The law is not an arbitrator of ethics; it simply offers a framework within which decisions can be made.

This chapter is concerned with how the dilemmas of medical practice in reproductive medicine are presented and discussed and understood by patients on assisted conception programmes. It is also concerned to discuss how the patients perceive them, and how the consequences are experienced. These consequences can affect family relationships not just in the present, but also over the life cycle of parents into old age and of the children from babyhood into adulthood and parenthood themselves.

Such an emphasis is in sharp contrast to that of medical practice, which aims to solve the immediate problems of infertility and involuntary childlessness. This is exemplified in how success is measured by 'the take-home baby rate': the consequences are for the parents to deal with and solve. However, it can be argued, first, that what the consequences are and how far they can be solved or resolved depend on what decisions are made or offered by clinicians during the course of 'treatment' regimens. Second, in standard medical practice the consequences of any form of treatment and its side effects are considered and shared with patients, before a decision is made to proceed.

Contemporary controversial areas are discussed in this chapter, to highlight the thesis that 'taking the baby home is just the beginning'. This emphasis on consequences is derived from research studies about outcome for these families.

The following issues are discussed:

- Ethical issues and dilemmas in IVF – biological parenting.
- Realities of multiple birth parenting, the dilemmas of multi-foetal reduction.
- Dilemmas of donor insemination parenting – biological and social parenting.
- Ethical issues of egg-share schemes – biological and social parenting.

The over-arching concept used in these different areas is the value and importance of taking a long-term developmental view in terms of the 'life cycle' of all participants. Disclosure is also defined within that context.

Research: what do outcome studies show?

Outcome research studies, which focus on the relationships in assisted human reproduction (AHR) families, are few. Snowden and Mitchell (1982) were the first to publish a social investigation into the practice of AID (artificial insemination by donor, later replaced by DI – donor insemination) and of the families created by its use. Their study was based on the records of a major DI clinic, where systematic records had been maintained about the referrals to the clinic and on the 480 children created by DI over a 40-year period. The follow-up part of the study was of 57 families with under-school children, and 11 couples with children over 18 years of age (Snowden et al., 1983).

A later study from the USA by Baran and Pannor (1989) explored the emotional aspects and experiences of 171 people involved in DI: recipients, children, adult offspring and donors. The authors used detailed case studies to present the findings.

McWhinnie's study (1995, 1996a, 2000a, 2000b, 2001a, 2001b) provides empirical data from the parents' perspective of learning of their infertility, attending a medical clinic and/or unit, and becoming parents after IVF and DI. The data collection covered both intimate personal relationships and the wider sociological aspects of family, kinship, social networks and the communities in which they live. The study recruited IVF and DI parents with children at different stages of development. Not a longitudinal study as such, it has provided data and knowledge about long-term outcomes.

How this was done and details of the methodology are described fully elsewhere (McWhinnie, 2000a). The rationale was that all the parents would have experienced infertility and would have faced the options available to them (continued childlessness, adoption or becoming foster parents). All would have experienced pregnancy and childbirth, and achieved parenthood. Once a baby (or babies if they had had a multiple birth) was born, what issues had they faced? Were there particular situations related to the *in vitro* fertilization (IVF) treatment and the child's form of conception? Which issues were the same and which were different for the parents of DI children?

The study consists of 54 families, 31 from IVF/GIFT (gamete intrafallopian transfer; in either case both parents were the biological parents) and 23 from DI, bringing up a total of 101 children, 74 from AHR and 27 step-children, adopted children or children conceived spontaneously.

The basic conceptualization was developmental, with regard to both the infertility process (McWhinnie, 1992) and the parenting (McWhinnie, 1995, 1996a, 1996b, 2000a). The latter was based on the recognized stages of child development charted through research and clinical practice by paediatricians and psychologists (e.g. Sheridan, 1973; Bee, 1981; Cohen and Westhues, 1990; National Children's Bureau, 1982) and the corresponding changing tasks of parenting in relation to each developmental stage (Erikson, 1959, 1980; Boulton, 1983; McWhinnie 1985; Kellmer-Pringle, 1986). Knowledge of communication patterns in relation to emotional, social and cognitive development and about children's understanding of abstract concepts, such as the passage of time, death and questions about 'Where did I come from?', derives from the extensive psychological, psychiatric and educational literature in this area. A child's particular understanding of substitute parenting, i.e. psychological or social parenting as being different from biological parenting, was derived from the retrospective life histories of adult adoptees, foster and step-children, and the considerable international literature about this (McWhinnie, 1967, 1969; Triseliotis, 1973; Raynor, 1980; Boult, 1987;

Brodzinsky and Schechter, 1990; Hoopes, 1990). A major contribution to the specifics of this understanding can be found in Brodzinsky (Brodzinsky, 1990; Brodzinsky et al., 1998).

In-depth, non-directive interviews combined with a retrospective life history approach were used. Both mothers and fathers were interviewed; they set the agenda of what was important to them and so were able to describe the realities of parent/adult attitudes, relationships and feelings involved in this new form of family building. The 54 families ranged across all social, economic and educational groups. The communities in which they lived and in which the children were brought up were equally diverse.

The study data were supplemented by interviews with parents where the children have been told about their DI origin, and interviews with donor children and with adult donor offspring, together with a search of the relevant literature. From these several sources, there emerges knowledge about the long-term consequences of these new forms of family building. The research study data particularly contribute to an understanding of a personal world where the conception of children has been achieved not by the eons-old method of sexual coitus but by medical intervention, either in a Petri dish or by the use of a syringe.

In vitro fertilization: biological parenting

The study of IVF families in McWhinnie's study, where all the parents were the biological parents, suggests that on the whole these parents could put behind them the stress of an IVF programme with its hopes and despair, and enjoy their children and being parents. All acknowledged tending to be over-protective or 'having to work very hard not to be'. They were also aware that they were 'the lucky ones', IVF having on average a 19 per cent chance of success (HFEA, 2001).

However there were continuing dilemmas. Most disliked and never used the term 'test-tube baby'. They saw it as 'a label', which might cause their child to be teased and made to feel different by other children at school. Many were concerned about whether to tell their child about their unusual conception. This was particularly so for those who maintained secrecy or who had been particularly reticent about their use of IVF and attendance at hospital. Ten per cent in McWhinnie's study had told no-one. They argued that this was a personal and private matter.

The dilemmas are also acute for those belonging to a religious faith or group that disapproved of the use of AHR techniques. Achieving a pregnancy and birth caused them ethical dilemmas. They had side-stepped their religious beliefs to embark on the programme. However, as they

were still active members of their religious group, their children's school-
ing and religious upbringing presented them with dilemmas and conflicts
of conscience. On the whole they opted for secrecy or avoidance. They
had decided that in a crisis they would seek out an individual priest
thought to be sympathetic.

As a result of early fears about possible abnormalities in IVF-created
children, paediatric and psychological follow-up studies were undertaken
from the outset. Van Balen (1998) carried out a comprehensive review of
these and concluded that there were 'no indications of a higher frequen-
cy of malfunction in IVF children' and 'that their cognitive and motor
development progresses normally too'. To what extent IVF parents are
marginally or severely over-protective of their children remains an open
question. Van Balen (1996) found no such evidence. However, it was
reported as an issue both in McWhinnie's study and in a detailed study of
mother–infant interaction by Papaligoura (1998). Papaligoura questioned
whether the greater continuing involvement that she found in previously
infertile mothers with their IVF babies, compared with those who had not
experienced infertility, could be potentially detrimental to the long-term
autonomy and welfare of the children.

However, it is noteworthy that all these studies concentrated on singleton births from IVF based on a rationale that the follow-up is to study
what effect if any the use of IVF has had on the child's development. The
comparative studies of Golombok and colleagues (1995, 1996, 1998) are
of singleton births for the same reasons, but also exclude children with
medical or disabling conditions. The reality, however, for IVF children in
general is that currently only 53 per cent are born as singletons; 47 per
cent of individual babies born from all types of IVF come from a multiple
pregnancy. The proportion of such births has risen dramatically over the
past 20 years (HFEA, 2001).

Multiple birth parenting and multi-foetal reduction

A review of the literature about multiple birth families (McWhinnie,
2000b) and the experience of the triplet families in McWhinnie's study
shows that the diagnosis of a multiple pregnancy may not be either 'a
ready-made family' or 'the ideal outcome to your infertility' as many participants on IVF programmes view it (Murdoch, 1997).

What is not generally recognised by clinicians or other staff on assisted
conception units, by participants on IVF programmes or by the general
public or the media is the reality of what is involved in parenting two,
three or more children of identical age. This was spelt out originally in a
major study in 1990 by Botting and colleagues (see also Bryan, 1992;

Denton and Bryan, 1995; Bryan et al., 1997). Botting and colleagues demonstrated the physical, practical, financial and emotional demands of rearing such a family. The crucial difference in multiple birth families from families with several young children is that all the children in the former are at exactly the same developmental stage and need the same amount of individual attention from adults as a singleton child needs at the same stage and age. An Australian study (Australian Multiple Births Association Inc., 1984) highlighted the reality and magnitude of the task involved. It found that simply caring for three babies aged 6 months and doing some household chores took 197.5 hours per week with no allowances for sleep, etc. As each week has only 168 hours, it is clearly a task well beyond one adult.

Added to this are the medical risks involved in multiple births – to the carrying mothers and to the children who are inevitably pre-term, and may have disabling conditions from this and birth difficulties. The figures show the extent of these: birthweights: singletons around 3.5 kg (7 lb), twins 2.5 kg (5 lb) and triplets 1.8 kg (3 lb); the risk of cerebral palsy: 1.6 per 1000 for singletons, 7.4 per 1000 for twins and 26.7 per 1000 for triplets (Office for National Statistics, England and Wales, 2001). Such figures demonstrate the need for hospital care for many of these newborn babies. Such small babies are slow feeders and require even more adult time and attention.

All the tasks discussed in the Botting study are time-consuming. Lack of sleep and exhaustion become a major concern. Finance is also a problem, particularly when the family budget had relied on the mother's earning. Fathers have to take on extra hours at work to replace the reduced income and meet the increased cost. As a result they are less available to help with the children. The mothers' social isolation from friends and contacts (even finding sharing care with other mothers of singletons may not be an option) results in greater reliance on their partner (Broadbent, 1985).

How do multiple birth families fare long term? The only detailed follow-up study of the well-being of mothers of triplets is of interest in offering a partial answer to that question (Garel and Blondel, 1992). The well-being of 12 mothers of triplets was monitored; psychological assessments were made 4 months after the birth of the babies and 1, 2 and 4 years later, with the total number of participants in the study at the 4-year review being 11.

At the 4-year follow-up all mothers reported distress, mainly fatigue and stress (Garel et al., 1997). Support from family and friends available at the 1-year follow-up had faded away. The stress from the incessant tasks involved in the day-to-day care of the children had been replaced by issues about the triplets' relationships with each other and with their parents and siblings. Their aggression was noted and was causing concern. One mother described her triplets as perfect at school, but at home she talked of their tyranny. Others compared them to a 'gang' or a 'pack'. This response and the triplets' aggression are also described by Bryan (1992).

Findings at the 4-year follow-up were:

- Four mothers required medication.
- Four spontaneously expressed regrets about having triplets.
- Three were able to accept the limitations of what they could do in the circumstances. These three had reported less psychological distress and more support from their partners.

Others talked of how there was no time to play with the children. No time to be with them individually: 'I am here to manage the practical problems and to maintain order.' 'We love them, but they have crushed us.'

The parents of the triplets in McWhinnie's study replicated the above findings. Delighted at the prospect of triplets and equally delighted with the arrival of three small babies after years of infertility, they had not appreciated what the years ahead would hold. Those who had coped well had an immediate family and social network, which was supportive and offered help without having to be asked. The parents had good practical skills and they worked very much as 'a team' in the care of the babies over the early years. What is significant for a general understanding of these families by clinicians and others is that only those who were coping reasonably well would consider spontaneously returning to the unit to show off their babies or to be interviewed by the media. For those experiencing difficulties, to tell the clinic would suggest 'we couldn't cope, after all they had done for us'. 'We desperately wanted a family so now it was up to us to cope.'

The question raised by these findings for clinicians, counsellors and others is how to present a picture of the realities and the potential outcomes to infertile patients who are desperate for a baby (McWhinnie, 2000b).

The response of medical practitioners to the so-called 'epidemic of multiple birth IVF families' is to advocate transferring fewer embryos. Studies done in the UK (Templeton and Morris, 1998), Sweden (Vilska et al., 1999) and elsewhere (Fisk and True, 1999) show that a good 'take-home baby rate' can be achieved when fewer embryos are transferred. At the time of writing it has been recommended in the UK by the Human Fertilisation and Embryology Authority that only two embryos should be transferred, although previously it was considered that three embryos should or could be transferred. This new recommendation, however, is currently being questioned. The findings of the studies about outcome are being disputed and exceptions to the general rule are being proposed.

An alternative medical option being offered is multi-foetal reduction, by which a triplet or twin pregnancy can be reduced to a twin pregnancy or to a singleton. There are medical risks: a miscarriage can occur. This is also clearly a controversial development. Is it ethical? Staff report that it is very traumatic and distressing for them. And what of the participants, desperate for a baby or for more than one, but not two or three or more at the same time?

Follow-up studies of the impact of this procedure (McKinney et al., 1995; Schreiner-Engel et al., 1995) have shown that more than 65 per cent of parents could recall acute feelings of emotional pain, stress and fear during the reduction procedure. Mourning for the lost foetus was reported by 70 per cent. Although most grieved for only a month, moderately severe sadness and guilt persisted, especially for an identifiable subgroup who were younger, more religious and had viewed the multi-foetal pregnancy by ultrasonography more often (Schreiner-Engel et al., 1995). However, it was concluded that most of the patients were reconciled to the termination of some foetuses to preserve the lives of the remaining ones. Much more detailed and long-term follow-up studies are needed to ascertain the long-term impact on families, their relationships and how they cope with continuing sadness and guilt. Reference to the extensive studies on the reaction of families to the loss of babies by miscarriage, stillbirth or when there is the death of one of a twin pair shows that such feelings of loss and guilt can persist for a lifetime, and can be very damaging to other relationships in the family. In addition, the impact on the remaining children could be similar to that already known to occur when one of a twin pair dies (Woodward, 1998).

An issue not so far considered in the literature is how far parents tell others about their decision to use this procedure, and if and how they tell their surviving child or children about the reduction that was done to give them a better chance of survival (McWhinnie, 2000b).

Donor insemination: biological and social parenting

In the three studies about relationships in DI families described at the beginning of this chapter, all the parents who had children by DI had opted for secrecy. Secrecy emerged as central to the functioning of these families, and their relationships with each other and with their wider family and friends. Such secrecy was maintained or 'managed' by denial of recourse to DI. DI was never discussed even between the parents in private conversations. Talking to the researcher was the first time it had been discussed since before the birth of the child (McWhinnie, 1995). Baran and Pannor (1989) described DI as a 'cover-up' for the man's infertility. They wrote: 'Most sterile men, who utilise donor insemination . . . do not deal with the emotional and psychological effects of sterility.' Such men are likely to be insistent that the child must never be told about their origins. In McWhinnie's own study, the interviews with the fathers frequently revealed unresolved feelings about their infertility, leading in some cases either to an over-concern and involvement of the father for, and with, the child or to a distancing from taking on a full parenting role.

An important aspect of whether secrecy is planned and maintained is that to the outside world this is a fecund partnership with children. The woman has been seen to be pregnant and a child is born to a previously childless partnership, perhaps childless for many years. If attendance at a DI clinic has been kept a secret, as it is in many cases, when will it be possible or easy to explain the truth about the child's origins? Experience shows that, once a partnership has presented the child to their family and friends as a child of the partnership, they maintain the secret. It is hard to turn back. How in later years could they face disclosing the truth – first about the child's conception, but also about the man's infertility which has negative connotations and which men frequently want to conceal from their own parents. They are certainly aware of the derogatory remarks other men may make.

The high level of secrecy is confirmed by other studies (e.g. Clayton and Kovacs, 1982; Snowden et al., 1983, 1998; Cook et al., 1995; Golombok et al., 1995, 1996, 1998). Studies have also been made of 'disclosure' rates, although they can also include 'intention to disclose' which of course may not result in actually doing it. The relevant studies have been reviewed by Zoldbrod and Covington (2000) and overall percentages presented: USA 14-29 per cent, Canada 30 per cent, UK 20 per cent, New Zealand 22 per cent.

A recent study from Sweden of parents of children from DI is of interest here (Gottlieb et al., 2000). The authors found that, of those responding to a follow-up questionnaire, 89 per cent had not informed their child of their DI origin, whereas 59 per cent had told someone else. Those who had told (11 per cent) together with those who 'intended to tell' represented 52 per cent of the total. The interest of these figures is that, since 1985, the law in Sweden has stipulated that all donors must be willing to give information about themselves to be stored centrally at the National Board of Health and Welfare. By the same legislation, children have a right to obtain this information when they are 'mature' – age 16 years. So the law alone appears not to have altered parental attitudes towards secrecy.

It has to be asked, however, how easy is it to maintain the secrecy? All parents in McWhinnie's study believed that they could keep DI a secret and that they could manage all that was involved in so doing. However, four mothers had already encountered the problem of being asked for details of the family health record. They had lied or given evasive answers such as 'Not as far as I know'. However, they realized that there could be life or death situations or serious medical conditions when they would need to tell the child, and were then faced with the realization that they had no details to give them. Other parents described incidents where they had to deal with many questions and comments about differences in appearance, e.g. eye or hair colour, or the lack of resemblance to the father.

Most mothers reported coping with these incidents calmly and with aplomb. However, there were exceptions, e.g. an older stepdaughter asked why her young half-brother did not have the right eye colour to fit what she had learned about mendelian inheritance in biology at school that day. Her stepmother was unable to cope with this direct question and fled in tears.

The long-term consequence of such secrecy is inevitably the deception of the child. The ethical question for the parents and for those practising in this field is: Can they justify this deception? For the parents, it is acceptable because for them the secrecy is about their infertility and that is something they consider to be private and personal. Whether this level of secrecy is justifiable in terms of the long-term well-being of the offspring is another matter. Also there are inherent risks to the serenity and stability of the family through unexpected or unplanned disclosure. The devastating effect this can have is already well documented in, for example, adoption literature, and in families where a child born to a young girl in the family is then brought up as if the biological mother is her sister and the grandmother is her mother.

Increasingly, DI parents are considering that perhaps they should tell their child or children, and some are now deciding on this course of action from the start. Many are influenced through personal experience of the devastation of children who have found out by accident about their adoption and the retrospective life histories of adult adoptees. A forum for this approach is provided by the Donor Conception Network in the UK, and by support groups elsewhere in the world.

One of the issues met by founder members of the UK Network was how to tell their children about their origin, what words to use, and what detail to give that would be understandable to pre-school-age children. Working with a DI clinician who advocated openness, two mothers collaborated to write and produce an illustrated book about this, entitled *My Story* (Offord et al., 1991). It follows the style used in adoption books for 4- to 5-year-old children and has acted as a valuable tool for many parents.

Where parents tell their children about DI, they find themselves in a no-win situation in the UK. As the children develop the capacity to understand what is really involved in their conception, they ask their parents, usually their mothers, about 'my' donor, or 'my donor father', what he was like as a person, his education, occupation, interests, health record and his family health record. Here the parent can answer only: 'I don't know'. These questions from the children are asked incrementally as events in their daily lives trigger their curiosity.

So it is in adoptive families as the children there go through childhood and learn about the inheritance of characteristics, eye colour, etc. from biological parents and in their biology and other lessons in school. Examples of relevant conversations about these matters in DI/IVF families are reported in 'What do we tell our child?' (McWhinnie, 1996b). Using a developmental approach, it shows the link between the stages of development that all children go through and the kind of questions and issues that can arise at each stage, what the child is likely to be currently learning in biology at school, the actual questions that adopted children ask and the similar conversations in the DI families reported in the text of the book. It takes this approach into adolescence and adulthood.

There is growing research interest in how parents negotiate the 'telling'. One such study (Hunter et al., 2000) looked at the experiences of a group of parents from the DC Network who actively chose to tell their child or children about their DI origins: 39 men and 44 women, of whom 39 were partnerships, participated. Many had found it was helpful to rehearse telling the child from an early age, using the *My Story* book; others developed a personalized version. There was concern about the possibility of upsetting the child and the child's reaction at later stages of development, e.g. the child being teased at school or stigmatized outside the home. Men in particular raised the worry that telling might jeopardize their relationship with the child. At the time of the study few found that their concerns were realized and overall none now regretted having told their children. However, it has to be noted that, as the children were of different ages when told, it cannot be assumed that that they all fully understood what being from DI conception really means (see Brodzinsky 1990; Brodzinsky et al., 1998 about when and how far children really understand being told they have been adopted).

Several studies spanning six countries followed up large numbers of patients from DI clinics. What emerges as significant is the similarity in the range of reasons given by parents for their reluctance to tell the child and which can result in a decision not to tell the child (Zoldbrod and Covington, 2000).

These are the same arguments that parents present when they say they intend to tell the child but keep putting it off. Reasons given for non-disclosure include: the child 'belongs' more to the couple if he or she does not know; the child might be socially stigmatized; the parents feared a negative reaction from the child; and the parents wished to protect the husbands' self-esteem through others learning of his infertility. In one study (Manuel et al., 1980) 41 per cent of the parents felt donated sperm was preferable to adoption in that it allowed male-factor infertility to remain confidential. These are similar to the deciding issues for the DI parents in McWhinnie's study and they offer a possible explanation for the findings of the Swedish follow-up study of DI parents already mentioned.

Would counselling before using DI have made a difference? In Sweden such counselling is mandatory before starting on DI and can continue over several sessions, but the parents can still opt not to tell. Without knowledge that they are the result of DI, the offspring will not be able to take advantage of the legal provision established with their rights and needs in mind.

What is significant about these arguments is that they are largely aimed at the protection of the infertile adults or partnerships and parent–child relationships. Only the fear of the children being stigmatized relates directly to them and to any concerns they might have as children and subsequently as adults. To date almost no attention has been paid to how DI parenting is experienced by the offspring. The prevailing secrecy of the 60 years of medical practice in this area has largely made these children, even as adults, invisible.

Very relevant, however, to any real understanding of the consequences of the use of donated genetic material is the life experience of adult donor offspring. What are the issues of importance for them? The secrecy of medical practice endorsed by legal provisions has made it impossible to make any kind of systematic study of their situation. Gradually, however, this is changing. A few adults have had the courage to go public about their experiences. By scanning the findings from small studies available and the literature of personal biographies in newsletters and elsewhere, it is possible to gain access to the experience of 90–100 DI adults. That number is continually rising as more and more are willing to talk and write about their life and experiences (Whipp, 1998; Gollancz, 2001), network with each other, appear on television and make a film (*Offspring*, released in 2001). More studies are also being published (Turner and Coyle, 2000), and their conclusions can be added to the growing picture of what it is like to be a child created by DI with its particular conditions for the child and their parents.

From the available data, there appear to be three groups in relation to being told or learning about their origins:

• Those who learned about their DI origins after a family disagreement or divorce, or from a step-parent.

- Those who were told on the initiative of their parents because of some other event in the family, e.g. a severe inherited illness of the social father (telling the child was seen as relieving them of anxiety that they might inherit the same condition) or when their social father died.
- Those who asked because there was something in the family relationships that had puzzled them for years – some evasions or some unanswered questions, or that they felt their father was very distant from them or that they were very unlike him. 'Perhaps my mother had had an affair?' For some the question posed was, 'Is it somehow my fault that I feel so different from him?'

No matter how they found out, the reported reaction was anger, resentment at the lies and deceit, and loss of a sense of self and of their identity. 'My story was destroyed. It was taken away. I felt I was in a vacuum. Who else knew?' (man, aged 46). 'I was not the person I thought I was' (woman, aged 44). 'I feel like there is a line drawn down the middle of me, and one side I know well, but where did the other side come from?' (woman, aged 53). 'We trusted our parents to tell us the truth, but they had been told to deceive us' (man, aged 54) (Speaking for Ourselves, 2000).

All wish they had been told much earlier; all want information about 'their' donor. Some want to meet him, at least once. It is a source of great frustration and anger that this will never be available to them, and that records from clinics and hospitals are not available to them – some clinics providing DI in the past have destroyed these records. For some, the quest for information about their donor father preoccupies them. The offspring wish it resolved in order to get on with their lives. A recurring comment about their anger and frustration is that no-one thought them important enough to keep records, and that the system was set up intentionally to deceive them and to make it impossible for them ever to know. Even their birth certificate is a lie. It says that they are the child of the parents who brought them up. But the father on the certificate is not their 'real' father in the biological sense. So how can they find out who their biological father really is? And how many half-siblings are out there whom they don't know about as well as uncles or aunts? If they are from the clinic studied by Snowden and Mitchell (1982), i.e. one of the 480 children mainly from the same geographical area, perhaps they live in the same village or even the same street.

If they have children, they too want details about the donor, his health, interests, etc. As the adult daughter of a 44-year-old DI adult said, 'After all, he is my grandfather. What can I tell my own children about him?' This illustrates the intergenerational consequences of earlier medical decisions in this area.

The kind of information and detail requested by children and by adult donor offspring mirror the questions asked by adopted children. A study of the adult adjustment of such children conducted before the now generally accepted understanding that children need to be told about their adoption and their birth parents and family opened up the area of communication between adopted children and the adults who parent them. This research (McWhinnie, 1967) showed that adopted people wanted factual details about their birth parents, but that they viewed those who brought them up as their real parents, were thoughtfully loyal towards them, not wishing to distress them, yet were themselves distressed when the adult world in which they had been reared had not always been fully honest with them. Some had suspected they might be adopted from stray remarks and innuendos from relatives or others, or from parental embarrassment at a simple question (McWhinnie, 1998a, 1998b).

The reaction of some donor offspring that they want to meet their donor at least once is indicative of the deep-felt need to have connections to kin and forebears. This is something adopted children talk about and understand (Rushbrook, 2001). They now have access to this information and to contact if they want it – donor offspring do not and are thus deprived of what most people take for granted.

The spectacular increase in knowledge about genetics and its impact on the individual's development and health history makes this deprivation more acute and unreasonable. This is so quite apart from whether it is acceptable ethically and morally to put parents in a position where they are likely to lie to their children or, to put it another way, to misrepresent the reality of the child's origins.

One of the many problems met by the increasing number of DI adult offspring who are talking about their childhood and growing-up years is that they have no organization to represent them. Two DI support groups, however, are providing this and campaigning for their point of view to be heard. These are Donor Conception Support Group in Australia and Infertility Network in Toronto, Canada. Under the title 'Let the Off-Spring speak' (Donor Conception Support Group, 1997) the Australian Group publicized a collection of papers, including 11 where DI adults tell their individual stories. The Toronto network produced a video of the first international conference on their perspective *The Offspring Speak* (Infertility Network, 2000). Further film, documentaries, video and written material are becoming publicly available (Whipp, 1998; Gollancz, 2001; McWhinnie, 2001b).

IVF with donor eggs: biological and social parenting; egg-share schemes

The discussion in the previous section was about DI, where sperm are 'donated' because of male infertility or other factors involving the male. Is egg donation different? Here anonymity is also practised. Studies show that, although women are more open in talking to others about their infertility than men, a considerable proportion of families created through donor eggs do not tell their children about their origins (Cook et al., 1995; Golombok et al., 1998).

Similar issues emerge as for DI families: when, for example, the child goes to school and draws a family tree, he or she finds other children and adults talking about family likenesses and from where children acquire particular characteristics. So the arguments about secrecy and openness are essentially the same as those discussed for DI families, although many will argue that bearing the child makes a difference. It does to the carrying mother, but not necessarily to the child, because it does not deal with the child's questions and curiosity about their biological background.

This is the kind of perspective, with its emphasis on the long-term consequences, that this chapter has emphasised. This should be borne in mind in relation to all current AHR practices; when new development is being considered; and new strategies are introduced to solve immediate practical problems. A recent example of the latter is egg-sharing schemes. These have been developed to solve two problems: first, the shortage of donated eggs and, second, the inability of some infertile partnerships to obtain IVF treatment because it is unavailable under NHS provisions in their area and they cannot afford to pay the cost of private treatment. Participants who require a donated egg and who can afford IVF treatment help towards the cost of those unable to pay, on condition that, if the latter produce more eggs than they themselves reasonably need, they will 'gift' the surplus to those who require donor eggs and who can afford the cost of the private care. Part of the agreement is that, if there are no surplus eggs available, the woman will still receive free IVF treatment.

Much has been written to explain the ethics and altruism of this practice on the grounds that the rules are clear and consent is obtained, and so it is not exploitative (Ahuja et al., 1997; Mostyn, 1998). There is considerable literature from donors about how they feel fulfilled in helping a childless couple to have the baby they desperately want, 'the gift of life'. Recipients also write about their gratitude. Although couched in the language of altruism and gift, it is in fact a form of barter.

The condition of the practice is that there is complete anonymity and secrecy on both sides about the outcome. Both sides separately receive careful counselling and, although they will be attending the same unit, care is taken to keep them apart with separate staff allocated to each side and their records kept separately.

The question that is never raised is: what about the children created by these schemes? If and when they learn the truth about their biological origins and that part of their story is that they are likely to have similarly aged half-siblings living in other families – possibly in the same area – what will their reaction be? The same of course applies to any children that donors have after their IVF treatment or other children in their family.

Experience with DI families has already shown that simply telling children how their birth was made possible is not enough. They ask questions about 'my donor' as they grow older. When they have siblings also from DI, they compare notes about their respective donors (McWhinnie, 1996b). Children in egg-share programmes will be no different. When they ask 'what was my donor like?' their parents will have to admit they do not know – although they had been patients at the same unit and at the same time.

It is now clear that many offspring find the fact that their biological parents never met hard to understand and accept. This will seem doubly so for children from egg-share programmes. Why did my parents not ask for information or meet the donor, who was in the same hospital? Why did no-one think that I might want to know about my donor and my half-brothers or sisters and where they are now? These are understandable questions. Yet they do not feature in any of the papers or commentaries on egg-share schemes.

The interest in half-siblings and the possibility of having contact with them is emerging in the growing literature and personal accounts of the experiences of DI adult offspring. Tracing has become possible with the availability of DNA testing and international networks and television. An adult who has made contact in this way with two half-siblings describes his reactions 'what doubts I have had about the profound significance of blood-ties, their importance in the story telling that is as much the stuff of life as the events it records, are gone now' . . . 'for me the discovery of these two has been like the warming of frozen soil after a hard winter, bringing growth and green into places that seemed dead and desolate for 30 years or more' (Gollancz, 2001).

So the questions likely to be raised by children from egg-share programmes who wish to trace their possible half-siblings will have a particular poignancy and irony: 'so near and yet so far', and now so difficult to find out about.

Discussion

Under the title 'Disclosure and development' this chapter has developed several themes. Disclosure has been broadly defined to include openness versus secrecy in relation to the origins and upbringing of children created when third-party gametes are used, but also to include open acknowledgement of the known and potential consequences of the techniques being used or introduced into clinical practice in this area. Development covers the stages of physical, social, emotional and cognitive development that all children go through, and this provides the context to an understanding of the relationships in AHR families. It also acknowledges the need to view participants themselves on AHR programmes from a 'life cycle' perspective. Using the concept of development means that one can look both forwards and backwards – forwards to the long-term outcome for each individual family created by AHR techniques and backwards to the previous life experience of the adults who become parents after experiencing infertility.

This chapter has covered the following contemporary issues, and raised the following questions:

- Do IVF parents need counselling and support to deal with uncertainties about talking to their children about conception outside the body? If so, how should this be made available? By IVF units that first provided the original IVF or by community health services?
- Are the realities of the multiple birth 'epidemic' fully appreciated, in relation to both the medical risks and the social, psychological, and relationship risks for the parents and also for the children?
- Is multi-foetal reduction an ethical solution? Do those who use it really understand the potential lifetime consequences – the risks and the ethical dilemmas it may present in the years ahead?
- In terms of donor births, is enough attention being given to looking ahead to the implications of this for the family, and particularly for the well-being of future children? Consent here is given by the would-be parents and the donors for the procedures. The offspring do not give consent, but it has a lifetime consequence for them and for their future children.

As far as possible, research studies have been used in this chapter in order to base the argument on empirical data. Additional data have added vital illustrative material to present the real-life perspective of the actual actors in these family dramas.

How are the questions raised in this chapter dealt with in day-to-day clinical and counselling practice in infertility clinics and on assisted conception units?

In relation to the multiple birth 'epidemic', the response has been to urge a change of medical practice in the number of embryos to transfer in one IVF cycle from three to two or even one. The social and psychological outcomes, however, have not so far been given sufficient consideration. One of the issues here is that clinicians tend to hear only from the successful and coping multiple birth families (Van den Bergh, 1995), whereas those experiencing problems are likely to stay away from where they were treated (McWhinnie, 2000b).

In terms of offering advice to would-be parents where third-party gametes are used, several clinicians are openly advising parents to tell the child (Professor Ian Cooke and Dr Sheila Cooke, personal communication). Others adopt a neutral stance, saying this is for the parents to decide. Whether those offering advice to tell the children also acknowledge, with the would-be parents, that they will have no information to give to the child when he or she asks specifically about the donor is another matter.

The evidence given in this chapter about the appropriateness and value for understanding family secrets that is afforded by a study of adoption research literature, the life experiences of adult adoptees and how adoption practice has developed historically is rejected by clinicians and some researchers in the UK (e.g. Shenfield, 1997, 2001). Shenfield argues that it is not relevant because one parent is biologically related, but mainly because adopted children have to deal with initial rejection by their birth parents whereas children from AHR are always wanted from the start. The contemporary consultation document on donor information also rejects the adoption analogy (Department of Health UK, 2001).

However, a full study of adoption follow-up research, as opposed to selecting a few such studies, together with social work and counselling experience with adoptive families and adopted adults, show that the separation from the birth parent is not necessarily experienced as rejection and as the universal trauma that is being assumed. This has been illustrated again in a recent study of the experience of adopted adults who have searched and had reunions with their birth parents (Feast et al., 1994; Howe and Feast, 2000). Also it is emerging that adult donor offspring can experience real feelings of rejection by their donor father whose attitude was that he did not even want to acknowledge their existence.

Given rejection of the adoption analogy, it is further argued that only when long-term follow-up studies are done comparing responses of offspring who have been told with those of offspring who have not, will there be enough evidence to answer the queries about the merits and demerits of disclosure (e.g. Shenfield, 1997, 2001). This is based on the argument that, until proven otherwise, the advantage of non-disclosure is that it preserves the privacy of the adults, the promised anonymity to donors, the confidentiality of the medical interventions and a continuing supply of donors.

The realities of carrying out research in this area (McWhinnie, 2000a) are, however, that parents willing to be involved in follow-up studies when the children are young, become less willing to do so as they grow older for fear that their secret will be revealed. Snowden and Snowden (1998) lost about 50 per cent of the cohort they were following up eight years after the first interviews.

The comparative studies of Golombok and colleagues (1995, 1996, 1998) also show a higher non-participation rate among DI families than among IVF, adoptive families and biological families. This is a difficulty recognized in the literature (Brewaeys, 1996). The exception to this is in follow-up studies of lesbian families where the use of DI has inevitably been openly discussed from the start of the children's lives. Here the participation rate is high and the child's point of view can be heard. It is not heard in the comparative studies.

The implication that 'telling' can be studied in isolation is far removed from the realities of AHR family life. The studies quoted earlier show that a wide range of factors and attitudes can trigger a question from the child or adult, and that this can happen at any time in childhood and also into adulthood.

It seems surprising that so much reliance is being placed on a project that would seem to have transferred the thinking derived from the methodology appropriate to a drugs trial or other clinical-type interventions to an area of complex human relationships and adult/child communication. The knowledge base is different; the methodology also needs to be different to take account of the multifaceted and developmental nature of the whole process. A reliance on such future studies before any decisions are made ignores the contemporary and immediate dilemma for parents and would-be parents. It also ignores the needs and rights of children currently being created by these techniques, and their welfare and well-being.

The question of the welfare of the child has by law to be considered (Human Fertilisation and Embryology Act 1990, ch 37, Section 13(5)). How this is interpreted varies, but is usually at the minimum level of protecting against potential harm from the would-be parents. This assessment relies on their past history and stresses child protection. An emphasis on the well-being of the children throughout their lives would bring this whole area of 'family building' into line with family and child care law, which has already established that in decisions in such matters the welfare of the child should be paramount. Adoption legislation in Scotland also adds the proviso 'throughout their life time'.

There is also an argument that can be advanced on the basis of aspects of the United Nations Convention on the Rights of the Child 1989. The articles relevant to aspects of the material presented in this chapter are Article 7 'as far as possible the right to know . . . his or her parents' and Article 8 'the right of the child to preserve his or her identity'.

Conclusion

Whatever law or international convention is involved to take further the ethical aspects of the practice of AHR, and particularly its long-term consequences, there remains a basic question in relation to individual cases. Whose responsibility is it to make sure participants and would-be participants fully understand the potential consequences for them as individuals and for any resulting offspring?

Counselling could play a major role. The provision of counselling is a mandatory part of the Human Fertilisation and Embryology Act 1990. The Code of Practice of the authority set up by that Act stipulates that three types of counselling should be made available: implications counselling, support counselling and therapeutic counselling.

The implementation of the 'implications' counselling has, however, become controversial. It is seldom discussed in any detail in the writings of British fertility counsellors, possibly because this could lead to direct involvement in assessment of those referred to these programmes. That function remains the responsibility of clinicians with the possibility of referral to an ethics committee in complicated cases. The actual knowledge and expertise of individual members of the ethics committee may, however, lie elsewhere.

The material and research data presented in this chapter lead one to a different conclusion, which is that the psychological, social and ethical implications for families should be based on a study of these potential consequences for that particular family. This would clearly fall within the remit of implications counselling rather than that of an ethics committee. Perhaps clinicians and counsellors should become more proactive and routinely include not just the implications of the 'treatment' process itself, but also the potential psychological, social and ethical long-term consequences with their attendant dilemmas. In this connection it is important that there should be a realization and acceptance by all health professionals, in this specialist area of medicine, that embarking on family building through AHR has all the hazards of normal pregnancies and parenthood, but also additional tasks and hurdles to be considered. This would require a major shift of thinking, from the current preoccupation with success defined by the 'take-home baby rate' to an acceptance of responsibility also for the long-term outcomes for the families, and particularly for the offspring, whose interests to date have been viewed as secondary to the wishes of infertile adults.

Annas, an academic lawyer and a long-time advocate of such a change, wrote under the title 'The shadowlands: secrecy, lies and assisted reproduction', 'The assisted reproduction industry caters to the wishes of adults, and their wishes consistently trump the interests of children' (Annas, 1998). In the same year a group of primary school children given a project to identify what they saw as their democratic rights built a boat to 'set sail their hopes in the next millennium', with slogans that 'grown-ups should protect us from all sorts of violence' but also 'children are just small grown-ups and we have rights too'.

References

Ahuja KK, Mostyn BJ, Simons EG (1997) Egg sharing and egg donation: a survey of the attitudes of British egg donors and recipients. Human Reproduction 12: 2845–2852.

Annas GJ (1998) The shadowlands: secrecy, lies and assisted reproduction. New England Journal of Medicine 339: 935–939.

Australian Multiple Births Association Inc. (1984) Proposal submitted to the Federal Government concerning 'Act of Grace' payments for triplet and quadruplet families. Coogee, Australia: Australia Multiple Births Association Inc.

Baran A, Pannor R (1989) Lethal Secrets. New York: Warner Books.

Bee H (1981) The Developing Child. New York: Harper & Row.

Botting BJ, Mcfarlane AJ, Price FV (1990) Three, Four and More: a study of triplets and higher order births. London: HMSO.

Boult BE (1987) Salient experiences of a sample of adult adoptees, MA Dissertation (unpublished). South Africa: University of Cape Town,.

Boulton MG (1983) On Being a Mother. London: Tavistock.

Brewaeys A (1996) Donor insemination and child development. Journal of Psychomatic Obstetrics and Gynecology 17: 1–13.

Broadbent B (1985) Post-natal care: twin trauma. Part 3. Nursing Times 81: 28–30.

Brodzinsky DM (1990) A stress and coping model of adoption adjustment. In: Brodzinsky DM, Schechter MD (eds), The Psychology of Adoption. Oxford: Oxford University Press.

Brodzinsky DM, Schechter MD (eds) (1990) The Psychology of Adoption. Oxford: Oxford University Press.

Brodzinsky DM, Smith DW, Brodzinsky AB (1998) Children's adjustment to adoption. Developmental Psychology and Psychiatry 38: 3–24.

Bryan EM (1992) Twins and Higher Order Births: A guide to their nurture and nature. London: Edward Arnold.

Bryan EM, Denton J, Hallett F (1997) A. Facts about Multiple Births and B. Multiple Pregnancies: Guidelines for Professionals. Multiple Births Foundation London.

Clayton C, Kovacs GT (1982) AID offspring: initial follow-up study of 50 couples. Medical Journal of Australia 1: 338–339.

Cohen JS, Westhues A (1990) Well Functioning Families for Adoptive and Foster Children. Toronto: University of Toronto Press.

Cook R, Golombok S, Bish A, Murray C (1995) Disclosure of donor insemination: parental attitudes. American Journal of Orthopsychiatry 65: 549–559.

Denton J, Bryan E (1995) Prenatal preparation for parenting twins, triplets and more: the social aspects. In: Ward RH, Whittle M (eds), Multiple Pregnancy. London: Royal College of Obstetricians and Gynaecologists Press.

Department of Health (2001) Donor Information Consultation: Providing information about sperm, egg and embryo donors. London: Department of Health.

Donor Conception Support Group of Australia (1997) Let the Offspring Speak: Discussions on Donor Conception. Publication from Donor Issues Forum funded by a grant from the Law Foundation of New South Wales, Australia.

Erikson E (1959) Childhood and Society. Imago Revised, 1965. London: Hogarth Press.

Erikson E (1980) Identity and the Life Cycle. New York: WW Norton.

Feast J, Marwood M, Seabrook S, Warbur A, Webb L (1994) Preparing for Reunion: Adopted people, adoptive parents and birth parents tell their stories. London: The Children's Society.

Fisk NM, True G (1999) Two's company, three's a crowd for embryo transfer. The Lancet 354: 1572–1573.

Garel M, Blondel B (1992) Assessment at 1 year of the psychological consequences of having triplets. Human Reproduction 7: 729–732.

Garel M, Salobir C, Blondel B (1997) Psychological consequences of having triplets: a 4-year follow-up study. Fertility and Sterility 67: 1162–1165.

Gollancz D (2001) Donor insemination: a question of rights. Human Fertility 4: 164–167.

Golombok S, Cook R, Bish A, Murray C (1995). Families created by the new reproductive technologies: quality of parenting and social and emotional development of the children. Child Development 64: 285–288.

Golombok S, Brewaeys A, Cook R (1996) The European Study of assisted reproduction families: family functioning and child development. Human Reproduction 11: 101–108.

Golombok S, Murray C, Brinsden P, Abdalla SH (1998) Social versus biological parenting: family functioning and the socioemotional development of children conceived by egg or sperm donation. Journal of Child Psychology and Psychiatry 40: 519–527.

Gottlieb C, Lalos O, Lindblad F (2000) Disclosure of donor insemination to the child: the impact of Swedish Legislation on couples' attitudes. Human Reproduction 15: 2052–2056.

Hoopes JL (1990) Adoption and identity formation. In: Brodinsky DM, Schechter MD (eds), The Psychology of Adoption. Oxford: Oxford University Press.

Howe D, Feast J (2000) Adoption Search and Reunion: The long term experience of adopted adults. London: The Children's Society.

Human Fertilisation and Embryology Authority (1998) Code of Practice, 4th edn. London: HFEA.

Human Fertilisation and Embryology Authority (2001) Annual Report. London: HFEA.

Hunter MS, Salter-Ling N, Glover L (2000) Donor insemination: Telling children about their origins. Child Psychology and Psychiatry 5: 157–163.

Infertility Network (2000) 'The Offspring Speak' Video of International Conference Toronto August 2000.

Kellmer-Pringle M (1986) The Needs of Children, 3rd edn. London: Unwin Hyman Ltd. (Reprinted 1992, 1993, 1996 Routledge.)

McKinney M, Downey J, Timor-Tritsch I (1995) The psychological effects of multi-fetal pregnancy reduction. Fertility and Sterility 64: 51–61.

McWhinnie AM (1967) Adopted Children: How they grow up. A study their adjustment as adults. London: Routledge & Kegan Paul.

McWhinnie AM (1969) The adopted child in adolescence. In: Caplan G, Lebovic S (eds), Adolescence: Psychological perspectives. New York: Basic Books, pp. 133–142.

McWhinnie AM (1985) Analysing parenting. In: Wedge P (ed.), Social Work – Research into Practice. London: British Association of Social Work Publications, pp. 67–73.

McWhinnie AM (1992) Creating children: the medical and social dilemmas of assisted reproduction. Early Child Development and Care 81:3 9–54.

McWhinnie AM (1995) A study of parenting of IVF and DI children. International Journal of Medicine and Law 14(7/8): 501–8.

McWhinnie AM (1996a) Outcome for families created by assisted conception programmes. Journal of Assisted Reproduction and Genetics 13: 363–365.

McWhinnie AM (1996b) Families following assisted conception: what do we tell our child? Department of Law, University of Dundee, Scotland.

McWhinnie AM (1998a) Who am I? Geneological disadvantage for children from donated gametes. In: Blyth E, Crawshaw M, Speirs J (eds), Truth and the Child Ten Years On: Information exchange in donor-assisted conception. Birmingham: British Association of Social Workers.

McWhinnie AM (1998b) Ethical dilemmas in the use of donor gametes. International Journal of Medicine and Law 17: 311–317.

McWhinnie AM (2000a) Families from assisted conception: ethical and psychological issues. Human Fertility 3: 13–19.

McWhinnie AM (2000b) Euphoria or despair? Coping with multiple births from ART: what patients don't tell the clinics. Human Fertility 3: 20–25.

McWhinnie AM (2001a) Should offspring from donated gametes continue to be denied knowledge of their origins and antecedents? Human Reproduction 16: 807–817.

McWhinnie AM (2001b) Families from assisted conception: How have they fared? Six families tell their story. A series of six videos on IVF families, Triplet families, DI parents and DI offspring. Chameleon Publications. Department of Law, University of Dundee, Scotland.

Manuel C, Cheveret M, Czyba J (1980) Handling Secrecy by AID Couples. In: David G, Price E (eds), Human Artificial Insemination and Semen Preservation. New York: Plenum, pp. 9–30.

Mostyn B (1998) Egg share donors and recipients: the voices of experience. Journal of Fertility Counselling 5(3): 14–17.

Murdoch A (1997) Triplets and embryo transfer policy. Human Reproduction 12 Supplement Journal of the British Fertility Society 2: 88–92.

National Children's Bureau (1982) A Job for Life. London: National Children's Bureau.

Office for National Statistics for England and Wales (2001) Annual Report. London: Office for National Statistics for England and Wales

Offord J, Mays A, Cooke S (1991) My Story (revised 2001). Sheffield: Infertility Research Trust.

Papaligoura Z (1998) The effects of in vitro fertilisation in parent–infant communication. PhD Thesis, University of Edinburgh.

Raynor J (1980) The Adopted Child Comes of Age. London: Allen & Unwin.

Rushbrook R (2001) The proportion of adoptees who have received their birth records in England and Wales. Population Trends. National Statistics 104. London: Office of National Statistics for England and Wales pp. 26–34.

Schreiner-Engel P, Walther N, Mindes J, Lynch L, Berkowitz RL (1995) First-trimester multifetal pregnancy reduction: acute and persistent psychological reactions. American Journal of Obstetrics and Gynecology 172: 541–547.

Shenfield F (1997) Privacy versus disclosure in gamete donation: a clash of interests, duties or an exercise in responsibility? Journal of Assisted Reproduction and Genetics 14: 371–373.

Shenfield F (2001) To know or not to know the identity of one's genetic parent(s): a question of Human Rights? In: Healey DL, Kovacs GT, McLachlan R, Rodriguez Hamas O (eds), Reproductive Medicine in the 21st Century. The 17th World Congress on Fertility and Sterility. Melbourne: Parthenon Publishing Group, pp. 78–85.

Sheridan MD (1973) Children's Developmental Progress. Slough: National Foundation for Education Research.

Snowden R, Mitchell GD (1982) The Artificial Family: A consideration of artificial insemination by donor. London: Allen & Unwin.

Snowden R, Snowden E (1998) Families created through donor insemination. In: Daniels K, Haimes E (eds), Donor Insemination. Cambridge University Press, pp. 33–52.

Snowden R, Mitchell GD, Snowden EM (1983) Artificial Reproduction: A social investigation. London: George Allen & Unwin.

Speaking for Ourselves (2000) Quotes from men and women created by DI/Remote Father Conception, Collection made available to participants at International Conference 'What about me? The child of ART' March 2000, organised by CORE (Comment on Reproductive Ethics), The Royal Society, London.

Templeton A, Morris JK (1998) Reducing the risk of multiple births by transfer of two embryos after in vitro fertilization. New England Journal of Medicine 339: 573–577.

Triseliotis J (1973) In Search of Origins. London: Routledge & Kegan Paul.

Turner AJ, Coyle A (2000) What does it mean to be a donor offspring? The identity experience of adults conceived by donor insemination and the implications for counselling and therapy, Human Reproduction 15: 2041–2051.

van Balen F (1996) Child rearing following in vitro fertilization. Journal of Psychology and Psychiatry 37: 687–769.

van Balen F (1998) Development of IVF children. Development Review 18: 30–34.

Van den Bergh (1995) Twins and triplets – personal experiences as a mother. In: Ward RH, Whittle M (eds), Multiple Pregnancy. London: Royal College of Obstetricians and Gynaecologists Press.

Vilska S, Tiitinen A, Hyden-Granskog C, Hovatta O (1999) Elective transfer of one embryo results in an acceptable pregnancy rate and eliminates the risk of multiple birth, Human Reproduction 14: 2392–2395.

Whipp C (1998) The legacy of deceit: a donor offspring's perspective on secrecy in assisted conception. In: Blyth E, Crawshaw M, Speirs J (eds), Truth and the Child Ten Years On: Information exchange in donor assisted conception. Birmingham: British Association of Social Workers, pp. 61–64.

Woodward J (1998) The Lone Twin: Understanding twin bereavement and loss. London: Free Association Books.

Zoldbrod A, Covington S (2000) Recipient counselling for donor insemination. In: Burns L, Covington S (eds), Infertility Counselling: A comprehensive handbook for clinicians. New York: Parthenon Publishing Group, pp. 325–344.

CHAPTER 8

Psychological therapy and counselling with individuals and families after donor conception

SHARON A PETTLE

Fertility problems are now known to be relatively common in the general population. In recent years there has been a developing body of literature on therapeutic work with couples facing infertility (e.g. Diamond et al., 1999). The Human Fertilisation and Embryology Act 1990 incorporated some requirements for assisted conception units (ACUs) treating infertility, especially counselling with those choosing donor conception as a way of creating their families. This counselling is particularly directed towards helping people consider the 'implications' of such decisions.

There has been little attention given to the impact of the experience of compromised fertility on later family functioning. An additional aspect exists where children have been created with donated sperm, eggs or embryos. The complexities inherent in such families (Nock, 2000) have not been the focus of research, although many social scientists have expressed concern about how the issue of sharing the information is handled. Whether shared or concealed, another party exists in reality, perhaps actively in the minds of some individuals in the family.

Such families are like others in many ways: they are not immune to the stressors of living, and may also face emotional, psychological and relationship difficulties, physical health problems, marital discord and divorce, unexpected death or other tragedy. However, some of their story will be profoundly shaped by their experiences around the discovery of, and reasons for, being unable to conceive a child naturally and their journey through to parenthood.

It is important to emphasize that donor insemination (DI) has been carried out in the UK for over 50 years, albeit unregulated and unregistered until 1990. The use of donated eggs became a possibility after the Human Fertilisation and Embryology Authority (HFEA) was established, and donated embryos have become available only very recently. It is clear that many parents (whether single parents, heterosexual or lesbian couples) who opt for gamete donation have given considerable thought to their decision and some have used therapeutic opportunities to talk through the issues both before and after conception. In the past two decades, a small but significant proportion of parents have maintained an open dialogue between themselves and with their children. The Donor Conception (DC) Network, a parent-led group, has been influential in helping others think about open communication. It is important to stress that, although this chapter concentrates on the difficulties that *some* people experience and the problems that *may* develop, these are not always to be predicted. Many families live with donor conception issues without significant distress, but inevitably the examples given here are drawn from families and individuals who have coped less well.

The 'social experiment' of concealment about a child's origins led to there being very little research available on which to draw ('social experiment' is a term used by Quinton et al. [1999] in relation to adoption practices that were initially developed without the benefit of any evidence and continued without systematic evaluation). Another consequence is that there are long-term studies in which children's origins are known to the researchers, but the children themselves remain untold. This presents a considerable ethical challenge. Families who have chosen to deal with this issue openly have rarely been studied. As yet, there is little evidence about whether donor conception leads to a higher or lower incidence of emotional problems or any specific mental health difficulties but some families clearly struggle (Hammer Burns, 1990). However, for those who experience psychological problems specifically related to this issue, these are real and often extremely painful, and present challenging dilemmas.

This chapter draws on clinical work, contact with many families in the context of research into the experience of being open with children and the narrative that develops, and on conversations with colleagues in the mental health professions. Some of the therapeutic issues will be outlined, clinical examples given and thoughts for the future raised.

Useful theoretical perspectives

Identity

New information about parentage is likely to bring into question aspects of identity. Theories about identity development, such as those of Erikson (1956, 1959) would suggest that the task faced by individuals discovering their donor-conceived origins late in life would be considerable and have many ramifications. This experience faces the person with the challenge of reappraising his or her sense of self and meaningful relationships with others, both past and present. Breakwell (1986) explored the fracturing of identity after significant changes such as the diagnosis of severe mental or physical illness, or widowhood. She commented on the threat such changes posed to identity and on the coping strategies that individuals struggled to develop.

From a social constructionist viewpoint, 'self' is created in language, conversation and interaction with others, and viewed in the context of changing relationships (Gergen, 1991). Thus, a person develops a view of him- or herself in the context of relationships with others, in particular from early family relationships and their place within the family system. The theory places importance on the stories we are told, and the narratives we develop to give structure to our lives (Sarbin, 1986; Weber, 1992). Relationships in any family are likely to be organized on the basis of available discourse. These will inevitably be influenced by a range of social, cultural and religious beliefs and values.

Using these ideas it is possible to see that doubts about origins might be conveyed in what children are told, or by what is left unsaid. The appearance of a previously non-dominant discourse (e.g. that a child is the product of sperm donated by an anonymous man) may have important effects on how people relate to one another. After such a revelation each person in a family may re-examine their experience, and the process of reshaping relationships may take place to incorporate the new knowledge. Therefore the family context is likely to be the place where many tensions are experienced as these multiple adjustments take place. Thus, therapies that place importance on the context in which difficulties develop and are maintained (both the immediate and extended family, and the social world in which the family have developed), and recognize the importance of the narrative created by the individual, may be particularly salient.

Attachment theory

A growing importance has been placed on the internal representation of the relationship formed by infants. The quality of early attachment is important in the later development of ideas about self and others (Bowlby, 1969, 1973; Parkes and Stevenson-Hinde, 1982). The coherent organization of early experiences relevant to attachment has been shown to be crucial for the development of security in adulthood (Main et al., 1985). The 'meaning of the child' for each parent is likely to influence how they feel towards the infant and growing child, and inevitably affects the way in which relationships develop (Reder and Duncan, 1995).

If one or both parents have unresolved issues about their relationship with a child and his or her entry into the family such that a secret develops, this could affect the attachment between parent and child adversely. Dowling (1993) pointed out that children are inclined to blame themselves when unpleasant feelings are not talked about. Keeping origins a secret might deny the individual the possibility of making sense of bewildering experiences. Without the factual information to explain rejecting or ambivalent parental behaviour, negative attributions of the self may be incorporated, with implications for later adult relationships. New information may lead to greater understanding and the development of a more coherent attachment narrative.

If parents have been able to create a secure emotional environment in which the child developed resilience, a later thoughtful and sensitive revelation might be experienced as less damaging. Alternatively, the concealment may be experienced as a major challenge to relationships that were previously valued for being close and loving, and assumed to have integrity.

Psychoanalytic ideas

Avery (1982) described the loyalty to a family secret as an inseparable part of belonging and hinted at the complexity of intrapsychic conflicts embedded in the family context. He pointed out that secrets both protect the vulnerabilities of individuals, and spare the family from challenge from the outside. He particularly emphasized the role of the family in child development. Using clinical examples he illustrated how the effects of secrets closely guarded by parents could be subtly communicated through mixed messages, and may be played out in the relationship with the analyst. He asserted that secretive phenomena might affect ego functioning, learning and the consistency of the super-ego. He implied that all families have some secrets, both between family members and between them and the external world. The question of what is defined as 'secrecy' and 'privacy' becomes very important here – because some boundaries, e.g. around adult issues that are not shared with children, or when adolescents confide in their peer group and withhold information from parents, are appropriate and do not usually create difficulties. However, situations where a parent tells one child a piece of information and insists that this is withheld from a sibling or the other parent may contribute to awkwardness in communication and artificially skew emotional relationships unhelpfully.

The systemic perspective

The differential sharing of information between people is clearly embedded in the relationship context. Karpel (1980) discussed the effect secrets have on family structure, particularly alliances and boundaries, and the implications for loyalty and betrayal, abuse of power and the potential for destructive disclosures.

In his classification, the concealment of facts about biological parentage would be an *internal* family secret (where at least two people keep a secret from at least one other). He elucidated the different positions in the 'awareness context', of *secret-holder(s)*, the *unaware* and the *subject* (i.e. the person whom the secret is about, who may also be the unaware). He pointed out that, although the secret might be framed as protecting the unaware, they were often created to avoid scrutiny, or to conceal a painful, or shameful, issue.

Secrets about biological parentage were seen by Imber-Black (1993) as 'toxic'. She stated that they blocked communication and damaged relationships, and affected healthy psychological development. They were seen as contributing to the shaping of dyads, triangles, splits and cut-offs in the family, and influencing closeness and distance.

Karpel (1980) discussed the difference between privacy or secrecy and raised the 'relevance of the information for the unaware'. He suggested a stance of 'accountability with discretion', in which serious consideration was given to the potential views of the unaware person, and that sensitivity was accorded to the timing and consequences of disclosure for this individual. Papp (1993) described therapeutic work after the concealment of biological origins had skewed relationships between parents and children, e.g. leading non-biological parents to be more distant, or parental ambivalence to be communicated so that the child felt him- or herself to be the source of inexplicable emotional and behavioural demands. She noted that some of the effects of unexpected revelations have been emotional distress, cognitive upheaval and issues relating to identity. Opening secrets should be undertaken with great care and efforts made to minimize the destructive consequences for individuals and family relationships (Imber-Black, 1998).

In conclusion, it is both impossible and inappropriate for there to be universal openness within families. The factors that need to be considered are the nature of the information concealed, the likely effect of this and later revelation. There is much to support early sharing of origins through donor conception, and to deal with the issue openly without it assuming unnecessarily large proportions in the child's life (Montuschi, 2002). Telling requires an on-going conversation that can be tailored to the child's emotional and cognitive development over the years, and responds to the child's questions as they arise (Pettle and Burns, 2002). One example of this process and the child's growing awareness and understanding of his or her own, and the family's, story has been well documented with children who have been adopted. However, it is important to report that the existing research on families who have chosen not to tell their children suggests that growing up in secrecy has no obvious ill effects when children are still young.

The context for families created through donor insemination

Discourses around the practice of DI have varied over the years (Haimes, 1998a). Reports in the public domain (Feversham Report, 1960; Peel Report, 1973; Warnock Report, 1984) have often provided conflicting views about telling children their origins and issues of donor anonymity. Clamar (1989) pointed out that the contract made between parents and donor with anonymity at its core has been supported by staff in assisted conception units but the child is not an active participant in this agreement.

Professionals who advocate openness raise the profile of the child's right to such information and the importance of openness about such a fundamental issue in the parent–child relationship (Landau, 1998; Speirs, 1998). The dilemmas for parents who had opted for concealment have been reported by McWhinnie (1992, 1995, 1996). Many described that even their daily conversations were influenced by this decision. To help parents convey information to their young children, books about DI such as *My Story* (Offord et al., 1991) and others (Schaffer, 1988; Schnitter, 1995; Paul, 1998) have been written. These have helped some families share the facts with their donor offspring, so that they, like adopted children, can grow up with the sense that there was never a time when they did not know.

Relevant research

Much of the research in this area has been criticized: small sample sizes, self-selected participants, the absence of fathers' views in some studies of children and parenting, quantitative rather than qualitative data and a lack of control groups for comparison have all been cited. Nevertheless, even studies with such limitations begin to help us understand some of these experiences and their effects.

The evidence is often contradictory. McWhinnie (2000) referred to a study in which hyperactivity was noted in a quarter of the children. Other research has shown enhanced psychomotor development and language skills. Emotional difficulties were found to be no more common in children conceived through IVF (Olivennes et al., 1997) but there was no suggestion that they were any less common either. Golombok and colleagues (1995) concluded that the quality of parenting was superior in families through assisted conception, whereas Hammer Burns (1990) reported that mothers of IVF children may be more over-protective, over-indulgent or abusive. Torr (2001) surveyed over 70 parents; many reported themselves to have had a distressing and anxious pregnancy, and many still felt unable to settle into being a 'natural' mother. These findings indicate that the relationship between mother and child may be affected in some cases by the impact of prolonged infertility treatment and the emotional toll that this has taken.

Although there is no suggestion that the donor-conceived origins of a child is necessarily the pivotal issue, it is an undeniable part of the family story and is likely to have an influence on how any difficulties are negotiated. In some circumstances, it may be directly relevant.

Harvey and Harvey (1977) reported that 90 per cent of couples said that DI had strengthened their marriage. Some findings have indicated that men may experience higher levels of stigma, which might affect the parent–child relationship (Nachtigall et al., 1997). The same study also showed that at least a quarter of the couples had opposite expectations about openness in the future. They found no link between the positions of openness and secrecy and bonding. It was evident (Currie-Cohen et al., 1979) that the process of DI was emotionally taxing for men, and particularly stressful points were the time of the initial decision, when the wife became pregnant and it became reality, and approaching the birth. The longer-term impact of infertility was studied by Hammer Burns (1990), who concluded that a child (by birth or adoption) does not take away all of the pain and marital distress. The group at the Ackerman Institute have observed:

> Couples rarely seek treatment because of past problems with infertility, as they are not likely to consider the relevance of their current difficulties to infertility. Instead they are likely to seek therapy for a variety of relational difficulties which may or may not be related to the couple's past encounter with infertility.
>
> Diamond et al. (1999)

Baran and Pannor (1989) powerfully exposed some of the real and painful dilemmas for families conceived through DI. McWhinnie (2000) concluded that, despite the limitations, if the research is brought together a picture emerges where, although children may be much wanted and loved, families are fragile when they have at their core a powerful secret about the child's origins, and that this issue is often salient in everyday living.

Adult offspring

Some attempts have been made to investigate the issue from the offspring's perspective. Snowden and colleagues (1983) studied families where at least one child had been conceived through DI. Parents only were interviewed and 11 of the couples had children who were over 18 at the time of the study. Contrary to expectation, several had been told of their origins in what was described as a 'purposeful and planned' way. Parents reported that they had told because they perceived 'that the children had a problem which could be alleviated by allowing the child access to minimal knowledge which the parents had about the donor' and their offspring had accepted their DI status 'equably'. The study did not explore in detail how this information was conveyed to the young people, nor was there any attempt to elicit the views of the offspring themselves. The brief description indicated that the needs of the offspring had been considered, and had influenced their parents' decision. The parents' willingness to be interviewed also implied that they had a degree of comfort in discussing the issue. However, Whipp (1998), herself conceived through DI, reported failing to contact any of the offspring, and questioned the validity of parental report in this context.

In their more recent book, Snowden and Snowden (1993) referred to a small group of young adults who were willing to speak about discovering their DI origins. Some were surprised by their parents' decision to keep the information a secret, and most were relieved that they had been told. They did not indicate that the relationship with their 'social father' had been affected, nor had close family relationships been disrupted. Some recognized the efforts that their parents had made in order to create their family, and as a result described feeling very wanted and cared for. It is difficult to assess the validity or reliability of this report, because the authors do not specify how the data were gathered, or how the sample was selected. No detail as to when or how the information had been conveyed was given, nor was there any information about how long the offspring had known the information before being interviewed. It was striking that the authors indicated that offspring were uniformly positive about their experience of finding out about their origins.

In contrast, a recent Australian publication of personal accounts written by DI offspring (Donor Conception Support Group of Australia, 1997) indicated that the discovery had been difficult, with far-reaching implications personally and in relationships. Reactions were frequently complex.

Some were positive about the procedure that helped create them, but expressed strong feelings about having no right to information that would identify their donor. Others were struggling with not having been told earlier in their lives. Many described the significant impact on family relationships, and numerous families found it difficult to communicate openly. Most reported difficulty integrating the new information into their sense of identity.

Information sharing

Research into the linked issues of secrecy and anonymity thus far has concentrated on the views of donors and parents (e.g. see Daniels, 1988; Mahlstedt and Probasco, 1991; Robinson et al., 1991; Cook and Golombok, 1995; Cook et al., 1995; Daniels et al., 1995; Lui et al., 1995; Adair and Purdie, 1996; Brewaeys et al., 1997). The reasons parents gave for secrecy can be understood in terms of shameful or protective discourses, covering up infertility, anxieties about societal stigma or a wish for privacy. Some parents felt that their child would need to develop sufficient maturity to handle such complex information. The majority of couples reported that they had decided not to tell their child of his or her origins, but a number had told selected family members or friends. Thus, the potential for unplanned revelations is raised.

Further considerations of different perspectives and possible effects

Biological parents

In discussion groups some women have admitted to feelings of discomfort during pregnancy after DI, occasionally to the point of fearing that they may be carrying a 'monster' or an alien. This feeling usually disappeared after the birth. However, it is not unheard for a mother, even though biologically related to her child, to feel deeply disconnected from him or her, especially if she feels that it does not resemble her or her partner, and therefore is a constant reminder of the stranger within the family. Unexplored this has the potential to lead to serious attachment difficulties.

Non-biological parents

Fathers who have not yet come to terms with their infertility or the use of donated sperm as a means of family creation may struggle with the news of a successful treatment cycle and the growing signs of pregnancy. The arrival of the child may not dispel these feelings, hindering the father from bonding with the baby. One potential consequence may be that the mother attempts to compensate and creates a dyad that excludes the father, compounding his feelings of being on the outside of the newly formed family. Attachment difficulties between the non-biological parent and child may be more common in sperm donation, because women receiving donated eggs will have experienced the development of the foetus. Mothers talk of subjectively feeling that the child became theirs through the process of nurturing and carrying him or her.

The couple

Diamond and colleagues (1999) emphasized that the process of infertility treatment places an enormous strain on a couple's relationship. How they have communicated about it, their openness with one another about their feelings, and the possibility to acknowledge and address conflicting or awkward feelings in the process of pregnancy and after the birth will affect the degree of strain that they – and the child – will have to deal with. In some situations, couples have separated shortly before, or soon after, the birth of a child. Others have lived for a significant time trying to manage the emotional withdrawal of one parent from their partner. This may also take the form of a significant decrease in physical contact between parents, one partner's unwillingness to be touched or, at the extreme, the cessation of a couple's sexual relationship. The non-biological parent may be distant from the child and become increasingly unavailable emotionally. If the couple's capacity to communicate deteriorates and they do not find ways to talk together and resolve their difficulties early on, it may become increasingly difficult to tackle the issues.

The birth of the child may resurrect conflicts around how each of the parents wishes to deal with their extended family. If left in abeyance during the pregnancy, this may result in arguments, splits and tensions, which may be impossible for the couple to resolve without help. Such concerns may also be little understood by those around them, who remain unaware of the child's origins.

Issues that emerge while undergoing treatment may be impossible to address at this stage when all energies are focused on the hope of becoming pregnant. Doubts can be very difficult to express once the monthly cycle of DI treatment has started. Thinking ahead to becoming a parent can feel like tempting fate, and raising expectations that might be disappointed. As a result, a host of new issues, or those that have been avoided earlier, can face a couple as they move through a pregnancy towards parenthood.

Families choosing openness

As yet there have been no systematic studies of children whose parents have opted for openness from the start. Informal contact with a number of these families through the Donor Conception Network suggests that the majority manage this information about their origins without significant disturbance – at least through to their teens. Whatever their struggles may be (and some do feel very strongly that they would like more information about the donor), these are experienced within the context of open communication and a trusting relationship with their parents. These young people do not face the need to incorporate such fundamental information about themselves into their identity at a later stage in their lives, or deal with issues related to concealment, betrayal and broken trust.

All children who have been told of their origins are not necessarily comfortable with the information, and much will depend on the family's attitudes and patterns of communication. Individual temperament and emotional resilience will also play a role in whether children experience difficulties with this part of their story and, if they do, how these are presented and how contextual issues are likely to influence the process.

> Abigail's parents separated when she was young, and she and her twin brother had always been told of their conception using donated sperm. Her brother Patrick accepted this fact with equanimity. Their (non-biological) father, with whom they maintained contact, made it clear that he did not want to discuss the issue with them and preferred that it never be mentioned. On reaching puberty, Abigail's behaviour became increasingly difficult for her mother to manage. She began to ask questions about the donor and expressed fury at being unable to know anything about him.

Parents can handle this issue with enormous sensitivity but, however open and supportive they are throughout, there is nothing they can do about the lack of information about the donor. Many offspring feel extremely angry about this, and a few direct this anger towards their parent(s) whom they see as having made the decision to use anonymous sperm donation. There are examples of this happening during adolescence where children have been told at a young age, or in adulthood for those who have been told about their origins much later in their lives. Some parents find it difficult to distinguish what might be part of adolescent rebellion and the move towards independence, and to realize how much this issue may become the focus of their discontent during an already turbulent developmental stage. However, the effects on the parent–child relationship may continue for a significant length of time, and some external therapeutic help might be needed to help resolve the difficulties, or enable all the individuals to tolerate their distress.

Offspring

There is a growing body of work looking at the effects of late revelation on donor offspring. Turner and Coyle (2000) analysed written narratives and found that the themes that emerged were: life as a lie/mistrust, withholding information and the effects on the family/parental dynamics, the need to know/making genetic connections, searching, talking/the need for significant others. They concluded that therapy would serve to 'explore thoughts and feelings in relation to their new identities'. They raised the importance of enabling offspring to re-examine their revised genealogical context and advocated the need for a specialized therapeutic provision. This might be equally relevant for those who have always been aware of their donor conception origins.

In my own work (Pettle, 1999, 2002), I have studied adults who had discovered new fundamental information about their parentage, including a number of donor offspring who had not previously articulated their experience. These people were not a clinical sample, but recruited through details about the research that were being widely circulated. This qualitative study explored in depth the personal experiences of 12 participants, three of whom were adult DI offspring (one male). All were informed of their conception using anonymously donated sperm in their teens or later. The impact of late revelation is strikingly encapsulated in one woman's statement (Pettle, 1997). She described it as if:

> the scaffolding on which I have based everything has fallen apart, but I don't yet have anything to replace it, I have to rebuild it.

On the basis of the analysis of the extended interviews with participants, a tentative model was proposed to map the process from revelation towards the integration of new information about genetic parentage. These six stages may be helpful to consider during therapeutic work.

Stage 1: the initial crisis – immediate thoughts and feelings about the new information and its personal significance

Participants conveyed that the revelation was experienced as an immense blow to their psychological world. They made it clear that their previous sense of identity could not be easily replaced even when details about the biological parent were provided. Many of the stories and interactions that had built the elaborate idea about self and relationships had been removed in an instant. The shock was evident even when doubts had been expressed previously or the content of the revelation was welcomed. This was reduced for the minority of participants when at least one family member was able to show sensitivity to them, and was willing to discuss the issue further.

Stage 2: reflections on deception and concealment.

In the process of adaptation, it appeared significant that others had known this information before it was revealed to participants and, thus, unlike an illness or traumatic event, it was not equally new to all concerned. It was important to trace how widely the truth was known within and beyond the family. Participants reflected on the times they had been actively lied to or deceived by those whom they had trusted. Feelings of insecurity and not belonging during childhood years were often reported, and from the data one could speculate that both the marital and parent–child relationships had been affected by the circumstances of the child's entry into the family. The child's perceived experience of not being cared for was repeated in adulthood, when feelings about how the revelation occurred again raised feelings of not having been considered. On the other hand, participants often made sense of confusing childhood experiences in the light of the new information.

Stage 3: deconstruction and reconstruction of existing relationships in the light of new information

Changes followed the revelation in relationships with both biological and non-biological parents. A greater distance in the relationship with non-biological parents (often fathers) was common, and frequently reflected prior difficulties. Mothers were often viewed as the source of the demand for secrecy, with fathers portrayed as being compliant. This sex bias may reflect the general expectation for the woman to be the primary caregiver and the implicit discourse in participants' accounts that they expected honesty about their origins. It may also have been that they were implicitly protecting their father, given their knowledge of his infertility and often explicit comments made about his vulnerability. The behaviour of people in response to the reactions of the participant (and vice versa) formed a complex matrix and affected future relationships. These were often made more difficult by the reluctance of other family members to discuss the topic, or acknowledge the impact and implications for the individual. As the person who was the subject of the secret, participants consistently indicated that they felt their feelings and rights had been ignored both by the concealment and after revelation.

Stage 4: re-evaluation of earlier experiences, creating explanations and giving meaning to the experience

Participants entered into a process of trying to understand the motivation for secret keeping and to make manageable what felt emotionally incomprehensible. They were often able to view their parents with some compassion, and as victims of the prevailing social and cultural expectations. Some could see that their parents' motivation had not been to hurt them, and indeed offered a degree of protection to them while very young. But it appeared to become increasingly difficult to understand a rationale that was to their benefit when secrecy extended well into adulthood. It became almost impossible when it was clear that revelation was never intended, e.g. when it occurred long after the parents' death. Significant relationships, past and current actions were all the subject of re-evaluation, and took on new meanings.

Stage 5: efforts to complete the narrative by accessing more details – technological information for DI offspring, the tracing and/or meeting birth relatives (where possible)

Participants were seen to strive to create a new narrative about coming into being and, where the identity of a parent was inaccessible, other aspects of the story assumed importance. For donor offspring this was often focused on the procedure or the place in which treatment took place. With the growing understanding and importance placed on genetics, accommodating the fact of anonymous donor conception was a challenge for all the DI offspring in the study.

Stage 6: explanations for secret keeping and revelation

Participants often gave a number of different explanations for why the truth had been concealed from them. The most common was the view that parents had considered their own needs at the expense of their children's. Social context was also seen as an important factor in understanding their parents' decision, and some felt that their parents were being protective of them. Sometimes individuals could understand why the information had come out when it did. When the motivation for this was not clear, they often described feeling as if it was a deliberately destructive act.

At present we can only speculate about the effects on relationships in families where open communication does not take place, but the studies reported here suggest that the impact of withholding such vital information can be significant, and the unexpected disclosure devastating. Although one needs to be tentative about making inferences retrospectively, there does appear to be some support for the likelihood that in some families significant attachment difficulties may arise.

Potential therapeutic work

Even among those people who may struggle with some aspect of their experiences with donor conception, it is likely that only a small proportion seek professional help. If the awareness of donor conception among health professionals was greater, the more likely it is that they identify those with difficulties and support them either directly or by helping them to make contact with an appropriate agency. The issue of donor conception may be raised in a number of contexts: at a primary care level with a health visitor or general practitioner, within both community and acute paediatrics, and in the education setting with staff at nurseries and schools. Donor conception may emerge as part of the story in child and adolescent mental health or social services, perhaps volunteered by parents or as a result of enquiries about how the family was formed. Occasionally parents may return to the clinic in which they were treated, seeking advice and support.

The nature of the emotional and psychological problems will obviously vary depending on who presents for therapeutic help, the nature of their difficulties and the circumstances that have contributed to them. Furthermore, the developmental stage of individuals within the family and in terms of the family life cycle will influence the dilemmas that may be presented, and which intervention is most appropriate. From a systemic perspective, we know that individuals and families may present for help with an apparently unrelated problem, and therefore the understanding of relationships and context is very important in bringing forth the underlying issues.

The therapeutic space (in whatever orientation) has the potential to allow individuals, couples and families to explore their story and find words for their experience and emotions. The importance of developing narratives to make sense of difficult experiences has been clearly shown (Harvey et al., 1991). This process allows people to tell, and retell, their stories, and eventually develop new and more constructive stories about their pasts (White and Epston, 1990).

Klock (1997) stressed the importance of mental health professionals taking a neutral stance and being non-directive about whether parents should share or conceal information about DI origins from their children. This may be too simplistic – people may benefit from access to such research as is available, reading relevant literature including that about secrets, and drawing on knowledge from fields such as adoption and child development. Then they can be actively helped to consider their position and potential actions. Professionals, as the holders of knowledge and expertise, should not withhold this from their clients. It is important that they are appropriately cautious about the research findings and that they explain to clients why the weight given to the conclusions must be qualified. Therapeutic 'neutrality' (Selvini-Palazzoli et al., 1980; Cecchin, 1987) clearly does help the therapist to remain curious and compassionate towards a number of different perspectives, and encourages exploration of different viewpoints.

Working with parents towards planned revelations

Helping parents to review their decision to conceal the information of donor conception origins from their offspring is likely to take the therapist into unfamiliar territory. So too will dealing with the consequences of late telling, particularly for the unaware or the former secret holders. Some parents may explicitly request an opportunity to revisit their decision, but it is also possible in some circumstances that the therapist feels that it is appropriate to raise this issue. Therapists should consider their own ethical position – and may wish to state this – but to be clear that a space to reflect is being offered, to allow the individual or couple to come to their own decision about the way forward.

Time will be needed to meet without their offspring (child or adult) present. It may be important to meet with each parent alone, especially if the parents are in disagreement or already separated. This is likely to require several sessions.

Reflecting on the past

Understanding the family context is important before the possibility of sharing the information can be explored fully. It may be beneficial to discuss the ideas each partner has about parenting and on their strengths as a parental couple. Inherent in this is likely to be their beliefs about non-biological relationships. Allowing them to discuss their views about openness and honesty generally, and about DI in particular, along with how they made their initial decision, is crucial to enable them to reflect on their position. Understanding how the secret came into being, and how it has influenced family life and relationships thus far, will also encourage reflection.

It may be very helpful to 'map' the 'secret system', using a family genogram (McGoldrick and Gerson, 1985) including the secret holders, the offspring and the unaware. It may be particularly important to include extended family and friends. Staff from the assisted conception unit, and other people from the past can be incorporated. Using this as a focus, discussions about their assumptions of people's positions and reactions can take place.

Exploration of the couple's experience of infertility, reasons, treatments, and quality of care and preparation will require sensitive and gentle handling: reviewing these experiences may be very distressing.

Help them to think ahead

It is probably useful to find out why they have decided to explore this now. In circumstances where the therapist feels it is appropriate to bring forward the issue of sharing information, asking whether there had been a plan, and how this was developed, may enable further discussion. Enquiring how they have planned to handle questions or doubts raised by the child, especially as they grow older, may help them face a possible reality.

It is essential to explore consequences of *both* telling *and* not telling, and to help parents consider the effects of both on different relationships: marital, parent–child and with members of the extended family and beyond. Referring back to the genogram may enable consideration of the potential for unplanned revelations.

The actual sharing

If they decide to tell, it is important for parents to think through who needs to know first. This may include preparing relatives and school staff so that they can be supportive to the child's questions. At the very least, this will reduce the likelihood that they will respond to the child with shock or disbelief. Parents may also like to create a support system around themselves to assist them in managing any difficult reactions.

Sessions can be used to consider language and voice tone, and the opportunity to role-play may be helpful. Explanations need to be age appropriate. It may be possible to explore the options of where the telling might take place, including within a therapeutic session, with the inherent support that this could offer. Finding a way of starting can be especially difficult and some families have found it useful to think of helpful triggers such as books, TV and news items. Once prepared, they are then able to take the opportunity when it arises more naturally.

During this preparatory phase, connecting with the DC Network, making contact with other parents, and having access to the available literature and children's books may help parents to feel less isolated.

What is conveyed to children along with the facts is important – offspring need to be given the message that they were loved and wanted, and created in the context of a loving relationship. It is important that they are enabled to ask questions, and that open communication is possible from then on. Adult offspring are likely to express a range of feelings, some of which may be very strong. They are likely to want an explanation as to why this information was not shared earlier. Younger children may appear quite unaffected as the implications of what they are being told are unlikely to be fully understood at that stage.

Given the complexity of the task, parents have to feel prepared to take this step, particularly as the outcome is difficult to predict. It is likely to vary with age – and may even differ between two children in the same family. They need to be ready for recurrent questions – or a period of silence, and accepting of distress, anger, confusion or equanimity.

Stressing the availability of ongoing therapeutic support, for them, and extending to others if appropriate, may help them feel contained, and better able to manage their own emotional reactions.

Therapeutic support for offspring who have experienced late telling

Individuals who have faced the experience of being told late talk powerfully about the lengthy process of readjustment that follows. Use of the tentative model outlined above may be helpful in guiding the work into different areas of the adult's experience. Both intrapsychic and relational aspects need to be considered.

If work begins soon after the revelation, the therapist's capacity to witness very strong emotions and offer a sense of containment through the client's sense of their self having disintegrated will probably be tested. Repetitive talking about the circumstances of the telling is likely to occur.

Once again, use of genograms can allow the individual to explore the secret system, and different people's places within it (Boscolo and Bertrando, 1996). This may facilitate a discussion of different relationships in the past and present, and how they might progress in the future. Such a process may clarify conversations that the client feels are necessary with family members, and the questions they wish to ask. Sessions that include others may be helpful. Some individuals may wish to redraw their family map in the light of the new information.

The aim is to allow the individual space to tell their story, and their experience of betrayal and breaking of trust, and to explore childhood experiences. These can now be reappraised within the context of new information. Although the validation of these feelings and experiences is crucial, it can be particularly beneficial to place the withholding of information within the social and legislative context, so that other positions can be viewed and considered.

When considering the stories of individuals some time after they have been told, the organization of communication about origins needs to be explored. This was important in the following example:

> Heidi aged 24, a postgraduate student, was the elder of two children conceived through donated sperm. Her mother had shared this information with her in her early teens. It was strongly suggested that she did not raise the topic with her father, as it would upset him. Her younger sister had similarly been told, separately from her, a few years later. No subsequent conversations took place with their mother, or between the sisters. As a young adult Heidi became increasingly uncomfortable with this position. A documentary about donor conception prompted her to ask for a consultation from a therapist with experience of DC issues, recommended by the DC Network.

She explained that she had had counselling while at university, but now wanted to think through the possibility of raising the issue with her parents. She was aware of the rift between her and them, and how she felt unable to talk easily for fear that they would assume that she was making an oblique comment about her origins. She clearly stated that she felt comfortable about her conception and loved her (non-biological) father as her Dad.

Beyond 'implications' counselling

The issues that couples may have to face when considering DI may be far wider than the implications of using donated sperm or eggs. Dealing with the diagnosis of infertility, and its psychological impact, individual, family and cultural perspectives on childlessness, assisted conception and the use of donated gametes, and consideration of alternative means of family building may be vital aspects of longer-term therapeutic work. This may mean that the sessions offered within the assisted conception unit are insufficient – or that some issues cannot be raised in that context for fear of judgement about suitability. Couples often refer to the 'implications' counselling sessions as a hurdle to be jumped over in order to achieve a pregnancy.

Another example of therapeutic work is given below:

Mervyn and Sarah were a couple in their late 30s in a stable relationship. He was left infertile following treatment for cancer, and received no psychosocial input to help him with the cancer diagnosis, subsequent treatment or with the implications of being unable to father his own biological child. Once referred to the ACU they accepted the few sessions of 'implications' counselling available before they embarked on DI. When they requested further sessions they were offered a meeting with a different counsellor – which they declined. They had no further support until Mervyn became significantly depressed and they sought help outside of the treatment clinic.

Mervyn's ambivalence about pursuing a pregnancy though sperm donation was very clear, and with some reluctance his partner – herself concerned about her dwindling fertility – agreed that they take a break in the monthly treatment plan. They were anxious about this, in part because they felt that they might be penalized by the clinic if they did not 'keep on going', and it was as if they had become infantilized by the medical process.

The therapeutic process allowed them, as a couple, to talk further about their sadness about not having a child that they created together in the usual way. It was possible for Sarah to articulate her feeling about the use of donated sperm, and openly acknowledge that she would have preferred to carry a child of her partner. Mervyn was able to risk sharing his fears about bonding with a child in the light of his distaste at another man's sperm being planted inside his partner. His African origins and the cultural context of his infertility were explored and the couple's decision to use an

African donor was discussed. After a number of sessions and Mervyn talking to at least one father who had children through DI, they decided to return to treatment.

Issues for the counsellor and therapist

The system that develops around families created with donated gametes is often very complex; at the very least it includes the donor and the treatment team. It is essential to be compassionate about all positions. Taking responsibility to understand the historical context and legislative context of DI treatment helps make sense of the strong drive towards secrecy (Haimes, 1998b). It is also useful to reflect on societal attitudes towards infertility, especially in the past and particularly for men, and to consider how sex differences may be played out in this area of experience. These wider discourses are important in understanding the journeys of individuals, and being sensitive and compassionate with adults who have opted to conceal this information.

The use of different language may convey more, or less, judgement. Individuals may have personal responses to emotive words such as 'secrets' and 'lies'. Listening to their language, or being curious about how they think about the position they have taken, may help the therapist sense how they perceive their experience. Words such as honesty, openness and sharing, or simply talking of 'choosing not be open', may be experienced as less pejorative and open the way for new thinking.

Given how painful and damaging unplanned revelations can be, the therapeutic context needs to be very containing, so that the process itself does not precipitate an 'unplanned revelation'. Parents may need support to resist the strong urge to 'get it over with' once the subject has been opened, and their feelings about it feel more exposed. Active encouragement to wait until they have fully explored the issues and considered how they might share the information with their offspring may be needed.

This may also be an issue for staff. The effects of holding the secret on a therapeutic team need to be acknowledged and carefully considered (Roberts, 1993). This is vital if this work takes places while someone is in an inpatient or residential context. A number of staff will become 'secret holders', and some people may feel deeply uncomfortable with this position. The danger of an unplanned telling may also increase.

Impact on professional systems

The power of the secrecy in the historical context, and the strong emphasis on this conveyed by staff in many treatment centres until quite recently, means that, within the therapeutic professions, little has been considered about how this issue and what arises from it might be handled. This lack of awareness may lead therapists and counsellors to avoid this topic or to bring to it fewer skills than they would normally have at their disposal. The following examples illustrate this powerful dynamic:

> A mother of adult children – one conceived by anonymous donation, the other by an intrafamilial sperm donor – wished to reconsider her earlier decision (much influenced by her treating physician) to conceal these facts from her children. When she raised this, the counsellor responded by saying this was best left and indicated an unwillingness to explore the different perspectives with her client.

> A young teenager dealing with the untimely death of her mother after a short struggle with cancer wished to talk about the information that her mother had imparted to her during the terminal phase of her illness. She had been told that she was conceived using donated sperm, and thus her father was not biologically related to her. Her parents had been divorced for some years and he had taken little interest in either her or her younger brother. Her therapist reacted to the information with a shocked look. The teenager was left feeling that she would be unable to help her sort out her feelings about this, and did not mention it further. The therapist did not raise the subject again.

> A treatment team in a specialist children's mental health unit was working with a family where the child was struggling with a serious obsessive–compulsive disorder. Parents informed them that their daughter was created using donated sperm but that she was still unaware of this. The treatment package was complicated in order to address family, couple and individual aspects of the case, but the new family worker was not clearly made aware of this aspect of the family's history. There were several important issues to be acknowledged and dealt with, including the couple's struggle with their own relationship. The issue of donor conception and the couple's views about this aspect of their marital story, including the impact of male infertility on them and the resulting relationships, were largely unaddressed. Consequently, their decision not to tell was not explored in any detail.
>
> In reviewing this piece of work, the therapist became aware that the information about donor conception was either poorly communicated or inadequately received. She considered that the strong drive towards concealment in the wider context might have influenced the process of therapy. She also commented on her awareness that had the biological relatedness of a parent been concealed through circumstances such as step-parenting or adoption, she would have been likely to deal with this differently and would have felt more confident about handling it.

Over the years therapists have become more thoughtful about the use of self (Real, 1990; Flaskas and Perlesz, 1996), and the need to be reflective about the prejudices and attitudes that might affect the process of the therapeutic encounter. Becoming aware and exploring personal views and experiences about family secrets, non-biological parentage, gamete donation, reproductive technology and infertility are crucial to doing work in this area. In addition, reviewing one's own position on children's rights – generally – and specifically in relation to knowledge about biological parentage is important. This area of work inevitably raises a number of questions about moral and ethical dilemmas, and it may be beneficial to articulate these, especially with co-workers, in order that differences can be explored.

The process of talking with clients presents a clear model that these are not taboo subjects – so reactions and questions are very important. Curiosity is a helpful position but it is questionable whether lack of basic information about relevant subjects is of any value. All the examples given here emphasize that the therapist needs an understanding of infertility, current treatments and the issues specifically relating to gamete donation. It is unlikely that clients will wish to educate counsellors and therapists about fertility treatment, and questionable whether counsellors and therapists can ask useful and sensitive questions from a position of ignorance.

It is clear that these cases may present at various mental health, psychotherapy and counselling services, whether they focus on services to adults, or children and adolescents and their families. They may also arise within health contexts and primary care. This suggests that this is an area that all professionals should become more cognizant of.

Implications for the future

The Human Fertilisation and Embryology Act 1990 proposed a Register of Information to be maintained by the Human Fertilisation and Embryology Authority (HFEA). In the future, adults will be able enquire whether the Register contains any information relevant to them (in certain circumstances this is already possible). They will have access to some non-identifying information about the donor and can be told if they are related to their intended spouse. Exactly what details will be given has not yet been specified, and donors have often left very limited information (Abdalla et al., 1998; Blyth and Hunt, 1998). This anonymity of donors adds another layer of complexity to the arena, as even parents who choose to be open about the means of their child's conception will remain unable to help them access the identity of the man who provided the sperm that made their creation possible.

There are clear indications that the recent media attention has perturbed some parents who have opted not to be open about the circumstances of their offspring's conception. This may be especially pertinent for heterosexual couples, for whom concealment has been a more viable option. Although the publicity may harden the resolve of parents who wish the concealment to continue, research suggests that some individuals develop suspicions about their origins even in circumstances where their parents thought it was a well-kept secret. Thus, young adults may contact the Register without having been told by their parents of their DI conception.

The shared ground and critical differences between adoption and DI have been drawn out, and it has been questioned whether sufficient consideration has been given to the position of the child created through the practice of DI. There has been a view in reproductive medicine that there is inadequate evidence to support openness and that parents should make their own decision (Shenfield and Steele, 1997). It may be helpful to reflect that over many decades practice in the adoption field changed from secrecy to a more open acknowledgement of the child's biological heritage. This change fundamentally recognized that the adopted child grows into an adult, and that the feelings, wishes and rights of individuals need to be taken into consideration. Adoptees now have the right to information about their origins, and a clear route by which they can pursue this. Post-adoption services provide a blueprint for how to proceed and pursue the wish to know more about one's history. They also offer support to people in the various positions within the adoptive/birth family system.

It would be reasonable to infer (Crawshaw, 2000) that a proportion of donor offspring will want to know more about their biological roots and wish to pursue this. Their inability to do so beyond a limited (and often very brief) amount of information may accentuate their emotional responses to the information, or become an issue in adulthood, even if as a child they accepted the information with little reaction. In addition, the development of accepted discourses about donor conception, late revelations and the process of integrating this information have not yet taken place in the UK. It is only very recently that assisted reproduction and donor conception have started to find their way into non-professional contemporary literature (Irvine, 1998; Zigman, 1999).

Given the historical context, it is not surprising that the level of provision of counselling for couples contemplating the use of donated gametes is limited. There is a virtual absence of professional psychotherapeutic services dedicated to understanding and supporting families who have used gamete donation, or for offspring created in this way. Given the possibility of changes in legislation in the future, increased publicity is inevitable. Many families may feel the need to reconsider their position and look for support and advice on how they might best deal with this information in relation to their child(ren) whose ages vary from infancy to adolescence. Families with adult offspring may also want to reconsider their position, even though the opening of the Register does not directly affect their adult children. Increasing professional knowledge and understanding of the issues related to gamete donation in the therapeutic context are therefore pressing.

References

Abdalla HI, Shenfield F, Latarche E (1998) Statutory information for children born of oocyte donation in the UK: what will they be told in 2008? Human Reproduction 13: 1106–1109.

Adair VA, Purdie A (1996) Donor insemination programmes with personal donors: issues of secrecy. Human Reproduction 1: 2558–2563.

Avery NC (1982) Family secrets. Psychoanalytic Review 4: 471–486.

Baran A, Pannor R (1989) Lethal Secrets: The shocking consequences and unsolved problems of artificial insemination. New York: Warner.

Blyth E, Hunt J (1998) Sharing genetic origins information in donor assisted conception: views from licensed centres on HFEA donor information form (91) 4. Human Reproduction 13: 3274–3277.

Boscolo L, Bertrando P (1996) Systemic Therapy with Individuals. London: Karnac.

Bowlby J (1969) Attachment and Loss: Vol. 1. London: Hogarth Press and Penguin Books.

Bowlby J (1973) Separation Anxiety and Anger. Attachment and Loss, Vol. 2. London: Hogarth Press and Penguin Books.

Breakwell G M (1986) Coping with Threatened Identities. London: Methuen.

Brewaeys A, Golombok S, Naaktgeboren N, de Bruyn JK, van Hall EV (1997) Donor insemination: Dutch parents' opinions about confidentiality and donor anonymity and the emotional adjustment of their children. Human Reproduction 12: 1591–1597.

Cecchin G (1987) Hypothesizing, circularity and neutrality revisited: An invitation to curiosity. Family Process 26: 405–413.

Clamar J (1989) Psychological implications of the anonymous pregnancy. In: Offerman-Zukerberg J (ed.), Gender in Transition: A new frontier. New York: Plenum Medical Book Co., Chapter 8

Cook R, Golombok S, Bish A, Murray C (1995). Disclosure of donor insemination: parental attitudes. American Journal of Orthopsychiatry 65: 549–559.

Cook R, Golombok S (1995). A survey of semen donation: phase II – the view of the donors. Human Reproduction 10: 951–959.

Crawshaw M (2000) 'Does he like doughnuts?' – the search for information about donors. Paper presented at British Infertility Counselling Association Conference, London.

Currie-Cohen M, Lutrell L, Shapiro S (1979) Current practice of donor insemination in the United States. New England Journal of Medicine 300: 585–590.

Daniels KR (1988) Artificial insemination using donor semen and the issue of secrecy: the views of donors and recipient couples. Social Science Medicine 27: 377–383.

Daniels KR, Lewis GM, Gillett W (1995) Telling donor insemination offspring about their conception: the nature of couples' decision making. Social Science Medicine 40: 1213–1220.

Diamond R, Kezur D, Meyers M, Scharf CN, Weinshel M (1999) Couple Therapy for Infertility. New York: Guilford Press.

Donor Conception Support Group of Australia (1997) Let the offspring speak. Discussions on Donor Insemination New South Wales: The Donor Conception Support Group of Australia.

Dowling E (1993) Are family therapists listening to the young? A psychological perspective. Journal of Family Therapy 15: 403–411.

Erikson EH (1956) The problem of ego identity. Journal of the American Psychoanalytic Association 4: 56–121.

Erikson EH (1959) Identity and the Life Cycle. Psychological Issues. (Monograph 1). New York: International Universities Press.

Feversham Report (1960) Report of the Departmental Committee on Human Artificial Insemination. Cmnd 1105. London: HMSO.

Flaskas C, Perlesz A (eds) (1996) The Therapeutic Relationship in Systemic Therapy. London: Karnac Books.

Gergen K (1991) The Saturated Self. New York: Basic Books.

Golombok S, Cook R, Bish A, Murray C (1995) Families created by new reproductive technologies: quality of parenting and social and emotional development of children. Child Development 66: 288 –298.

Hammer Burns L (1990) An exploratory study of perceptions of parenting after infertility. Family Systems Medicine 8: 177–189.

Haimes E (1998a) The making of 'the DI child': changing representations of people conceived through donor insemination. In: Daniels KR, Haimes E (eds), Donor Insemination. International social science perspectives. Cambridge: Cambridge University Press, pp. 53–75.

Haimes E (1998b) Truth and the child: a sociological perspective. In Blyth E, Crawshaw M, Speirs J (eds),Truth and the Child 10 Years On: Information exchange in donor-assisted conception. Birmingham: British Association of Social Workers, pp. 5–8.

Harvey B, Harvey A (1977) How couples feel about donor insemination. Contemporary Obstetrics and Gynaecology 9: 10–17.

Harvey JH, Orbuch TL, Chwalisz KD, Garwood G (1991) Coping with sexual assault: the roles of account-making and confiding. Journal of Traumatic Stress 4: 515–531.

Imber-Black E (ed.) (1993) Secrets in Families and Family Therapy. New York: WW Norton.

Imber-Black E (1998) The Secret Life of Families. How secrets shape relationships – when and how to tell. London: Thorsons.

Irvine J (1998) A Widow for One Year. London: Bloomsbury.

Karpel MA (1980) Family Secrets: i. Conceptual and ethical issues in the relational context, ii. Ethical and practical considerations in therapeutic management. Family Process 19: 295–306.

Klock SC (1997) The controversy surrounding privacy or disclosure among donor gamete recipients. Journal of Assisted Reproduction and Genetics 14: 378–380.

Landau R (1998) The management of genetic origins: secrecy and openness in donor assisted conception in Israel and elsewhere. Human Reproduction 13: 3268–3273.

Lui SC, Weaver SM, Robinson J et al. (1995) A survey of semen donor attitudes. Human Reproduction 10: 234–238.

McGoldrick M, Gerson R (1985) Genograms in Family Assessment. New York: Norton.

McWhinnie AM (1992) Creating children: the medical and social dilemmas of assisted reproduction. Early Child Development and Care 81: 39–54.

McWhinnie AM (1995) A study of parenting of IVF and DI children: the social and legal dilemmas. International Journal of Medicine and the Law 14(7/8): 501–508.

McWhinnie AM (1996) Families following assisted conception. What do we tell our child? Department of Social Work, University of Dundee.

McWhinnie AM (2000) Children from assisted reproductive technology: the psychological issues and ethical dilemmas. Early Child Development and Care 163: 13–23.

Mahlstedt PP, Probasco A (1991) Sperm donors: their attitudes towards providing medical and psychosocial information for recipient couples and donor offspring. Infertility and Sterility 56: 747–753.

Main M, Kaplan N, Cassidy J (1985) Security in infancy, childhood and adulthood: a move to the level of representation. In Bretherton I, Waters E (eds), Growing Points of Attachment Theory and Research. Monographs of the Society for Research into Child Development, 50 (1–2, Serial No. 209), pp. 66–104.

Montuschi O (2002) Support and information needs of parents with children conceived through assisted conception. In: Nolan M (ed.), Education and Support for Parenting – A Guide for Health Professionals. London: Churchill Livingstone, Chapter 12.

Nachtigall RD, Tschann JM, Szkupinski Quiroga S, Pitcher L, Becker G (1997) Stigma, disclosure and family functioning among parents of children conceived through donor insemination. Fertility and Sterility 68: 83–89.

Nock SL (2000) The divorce of marriage and parenthood. Journal of Family Therapy 22: 245 – 263.

Offord J, Mays A, Cooke S (1991) My Story (revised 2001). Sheffield: Infertility Research Trust.

Olivennes F, Kerbrat V, Rufat P, Blanchet V, Fanchin R, Frydman R (1997) Follow up of a cohort of 422 children aged 6 to 13 years conceived by in vitro fertilisation. Fertility and Sterility 67: 284–289.

Papp P (1993) The worm in the bud: secrets between parents and children. In: Imber-Black E (ed.), Secrets in Families and Family Therapy. New York: WW Norton, pp 66–85.

Parkes CM, Stevenson-Hinde J (eds) (1982) The Place of Attachment in Human Behaviour. London: Tavistock.

Paul J (1988) How I Began: The story of donor insemination. Victoria, Australia: Ambassador Press.

Peel Report (1973) Report of the Panel on Human Artificial Insemination. British Medical Journal ii(suppl): 3–5.

Pettle SA (1997) An exploration of the impact of the disclosure of information regarding biological parentage using semi-structured interviews, genograms and repertory grid technique. Unpublished research report. Salomons/Canterbury Christ Church College.

Pettle SA (1999) Secrets about biological parentage: a qualitative study. Unpublished doctoral thesis. Salomons/Canterbury Christ Church University College.

Pettle SA (2002) Some findings from research into secrets about biological parentage. The Magazine for Family Therapy and Systemic Practice. Special edn, Researching Families and Family Therapy 2–4.

Pettle SA, Burns J (2002) Choosing to be open about donor conception: the experiences of parents. London: Donor Conception Network.

Quinton D, Selwyn J, Rushton A, Dance C (1999) Contact between children placed away from home and their birth parents: Ryburn's 'reanalysis' analysed. Clinical Child Psychology and Psychiatry 4: 519–531.

Real T (1990) The therapeutic use of self in constructionist systemic therapy. Family Process 29: 255–272.

Reder P, Duncan S (1995) The meaning of the child. In: Reder P, Lucey C (eds), Assessment of Parenting. Psychiatric and Psychological Contributions. London: Routledge, pp. 39–55.

Roberts J (1993) On trainees and training: safety, secrets and revelation. In: Imber-Black E (ed) Secrets in Families and Family Therapy. New York: WW Norton, pp. 389–410.

Robinson JN, Forman RG, Clark AM, Egan DM, Chapman MG, Barlow DH (1991) Attitudes of donors and recipients to gamete donation. Human Reproduction 6: 307–309.

Sarbin TR (ed.) (1986) Narrative Psychology: The storied nature of human conduct. New York: Praeger.

Schaffer P (1988) How Babies and Families are Made: (There is more than one way!). Berkeley, Calif: Tabor Sarah Books.

Schnitter JT (1995) Let Me Explain. A story about donor insemination. Indianapolis: Perspectives Press.

Selvini-Palazzoli M, Boscolo L, Cecchin G, Prata G (1980) Hypothesizing–circularity–neutrality: three guidelines for the conductor of the session. Family Process 19: 3–12.

Shenfield F, Steele SJ (1997) What are the effects of anonymity and secrecy on the welfare of the child in gamete donation? Human Reproduction 12: 392 – 395.

Snowden R, Snowden E (1993) The Gift of a Child, 2nd edn. Exeter: University of Exeter Press.

Snowden R, Mitchell GD, Snowden EM (1983) Artificial Reproduction: A social investigation. London: Allen & Unwin.

Speirs J (1998) Children's rights or adults' rights? In: Blyth E, Crawshaw M, Speirs J (eds), Truth and the Child 10 Years On: Information exchange in donor-assisted conception. Birmingham: British Association of Social Workers, pp. 15–22.

Torr H (2001) The Experience of Pregnancy and Parenthood after Assisted Conception. A survey. Nottingham: AceBabes.

Turner AJ, Coyle A (2000) What does it mean to be a donor offspring? The identity experiences of adults conceived by donor insemination and the implications for counselling and therapy. Human Reproduction 15: 2041–2051.

Warnock Report (1984) Department of Health and Social Security Report of the Committee of Inquiry into Human Fertilisation and Embryology. Cmnd 9414. London: HMSO.

Weber AL (1992) The account-making process: a phenomenological approach. In: Orbuch, TL (ed.), Close Relationship Loss. New York: Springer Verlag, pp. 174–191.

Whipp C (1998) The legacy of deceit: a donor offspring's perspective on secrecy in assisted conception. In: Blyth E, Crawshaw M, Speirs J (eds), Truth and the Child 10 Years On: Information exchange in donor-assisted conception. Birmingham: British Association of Social Workers, pp. 61–64.

White M, Epston D (1990) Narrative Means to Therapeutic Ends. New York: WW Norton.

Zigman L (1999) Dating Big Bird. London: Hutchinson.

CHAPTER 9

Policy development in third-party reproduction: an international perspective

KEN DANIELS

In a recent Australian television documentary 17-year-old Geraldine Hewitt said:

> I certainly haven't missed out on having a great family but I definitely will be maintaining my search for the donor, it's not vital in terms of my being a well-rounded human being but I think that it's an extremely important part of my finding my own sense of identity and place in the world. I think it's extremely important for my children because they too will have 25% of their medical history missing and I have no idea what kind of hereditary diseases I might inherit. I think that these people who are trying to enact laws to govern part of the medical technologies of today and the future they really do have to focus their attention on the people who's [sic] lives they are actually playing around with – the donor offspring.
>
> Hewitt (2001)

At virtually the same time, Television New Zealand produced a documentary focusing on the experiences of Rebecca Hamilton, a 23-year-old student who is searching to find the person who had contributed semen for her parents. Rebecca's moving and at times very painful journey was being undertaken because of her need to have more information about her genetic background. Her widowed mother who also took part in the programme was fully supportive of Rebecca's endeavours (Hamilton, 2001).

As Susannah Merricks, who is 14, and lives in the UK has said:

> Tracing my donor is something I am definitely going to try to do. It's very hard growing up and not knowing the other side of your genetic background and also dangerous if there is a history of family diseases. It's not that I feel deceived or let down by the medical profession but I don't feel complete and at the least I want to know what colour eyes my donor has.

As much as I get all the love and support I need at home, it really upsets me when people say things like I have my father's nose and my mother's mouth, as they don't realize how special it is just to say that. When you know which bits of you came from your mum and your dad, then you can focus on who you are. Trying to figure that out is hard enough let alone being a DI child and only knowing half. Knowing could establish what is what and help me feel relaxed and secure.

My father is 100 per cent Walter Merricks – the person who has been there since the day I was born, the man who wants me as his daughter, the man who loves me with all his heart, the man who has always been there for me and always will be. In no way would I ever consider my donor as my father.

Walters (2000)

Bill Cordray, a 54-year-old American (conceived as a result of DI), has been a central figure in the call for a change in the way in which donor insemination (DI) is practised and in particular the anonymity of the man providing his semen.

We trusted our parents to tell us the truth, but they had been told to deceive us. We looked for information from doctors who had sworn an oath to do no harm, but they had destroyed our medical records. We hoped for understanding of our emotional experiences from social scientists and psychologists, but they encountered a wall of secrecy that prevented them from studying us, or else they studied us as small children and proclaimed that they could see no problems at all.

As adult citizens, we asked for justice and equal protection of our rights by governments and the courts, but they placed legal barriers in our way to prevent us from knowing who we are.

How long can this go on? When will we earn the rights of ordinary citizens to know our identity, our sense of ancestral heritage? We are left to make sense of ourselves without the roadmap of our genetic blueprint. We are lost in an unfamiliar landscape. We are invisible.

Cordray (personal communication)

These four examples from four different countries represent perhaps the most significant and dramatic challenge to the way in which the policy and practice of third-party reproduction has been practised. All four of these individuals are extremely grateful that their parents used DI and, as a result, they were born. Their concerns centre on the fact that at the time the decisions were being made about the use of DI, insufficient attention was given to recognizing what their needs might be, especially in later life. This was because the decision-making was in the hands of health professionals – in particular doctors – and their parents. Their parents reported, however, that they were very dependent on the doctors for advice and guidance. In all four situations, information about the man who provided his semen was not recorded or is now not available, or there has been a refusal to pass on such information.

Legislation has been introduced in Sweden (Swedish Law on Artificial Insemination 1985), Austria (Federal Law on Medically Assisted Procreation 1992), the State of Victoria, Australia (Infertility Treatment Act 1998) and Switzerland (Federal Law on Medically Assisted Reproduction 1998, updated 2001) to ensure that appropriate records are now maintained and that offspring, when they reach an appropriate age, will be able to access information about their background and possibly make contact with the semen provider should they wish to. In the Netherlands, it will soon become compulsory by law to register the gamete provider's identity (Brewaeys, 2001). These five jurisdictions have recognized that the experiences of the four people mentioned above have social as well as personal consequences, and their introduction of legislation has acknowledged that the rights of the offspring need to be recognized and protected as a matter of public policy.

This chapter, with its focus on policy development, maps the way in which the 'private troubles' of offspring, born as a result of third-party reproduction (such as Geraldine, Rebecca, Susannah and Bill), and indeed their parents and the gamete providers, are being increasingly seen as a 'public issue' (Mills, 1970). Public issues invariably lead to public policy. Anderson (1990) has pointed out that there are five stages in the process of policy development: problem identification and agenda setting, policy formation, policy adoption, policy implementation and policy evaluation.

There has been a growing recognition, mainly since the birth of Louise Brown after *in vitro* fertilization (IVF) treatment in 1978, that issues associated with assisted human reproduction (AHR) demand public consideration and response. In Anderson's model, problem identification has taken place and, in many jurisdictions that has been as far as matters have progressed. The setting of an agenda and policy formation has been much more problematic, because they require resolution of conflicting perspectives. Some jurisdictions, however, have not only formulated policies, but also gone on to adopt and implement them, examples being the countries cited above. This is not to suggest that the policy, once adopted, remains static because those who, for whatever reason, are unhappy with the policy will wish to challenge it and call for review. New evidence and information may also lead to a questioning of existing policy. This is sometimes associated with the stage of policy evaluation in which some parties question whether the policy is achieving what it was designed to achieve.

This chapter considers the move to a public policy perspective in third-party reproduction and then explores the issues and implications of information sharing in third-party reproduction. This exploration will focus on the interests of the offspring and their families, and the gamete providers. Throughout, reference will be made to the role of the professionals – in particular doctors – as the gatekeepers and managers of information sharing. The literature cited is, in the main, drawn from the field of DI, because of its longer history and because the culture of secrecy was established around DI. The chapter does not include a discussion of embryo donation, surrogacy or IVF, although many of the issues raised apply to or can be generalized to these areas of AHR.

From private ordering to public policy

In his deeply disturbing book, *Blizzard and the Holy Ghost* (1977), Joseph Blizzard (a doctor) says: 'Over the past twenty five years AID [artificial insemination by donor] has not been a very prominent issue. It is practised in a quiet and almost furtive manner. ' Blizzard felt that he and his wife were subjected to inappropriate and unhelpful treatment from his fellow doctors as they sought and used DI. Blizzard says, 'the issue which chiefly concerns me is [that] the climate of conspiracy surrounding the practice of AID seems almost deliberately designed to compromise the interest of those who might in clearer circumstances, be considered its beneficiaries' (Blizzard, 1977, pp. 18, 19). It is primarily a concern for the participants in DI and especially the children/offspring that has led to the placing of this procedure on the public agenda. Throughout this chapter, the term 'offspring' is used, because the term 'child' is inappropriate when discussing adults conceived as a result of DI. It should also be noted that the use of the term 'child' tends to lead to notions of paternalism and protection (Rowland, 1984), and such notions are firmly rejected by people such as Geraldine, Rebecca, Susannah and Bill.

Addison Hard reported the first case of DI using human semen, in 1909:

Hard was a student of Dr William Pancoast who, while teaching a class at Jefferson Medical College in 1884, discussed a situation in which the male in a couple was discovered to be azoospermic and the female was found to be capable of bearing children. The students in this class suggested that a 'hired man' be called in to solve the problem. Dr Pancoast then took a semen sample from the 'best looking member of the class' and inseminated the woman without her consent and while she was anaesthetized. The doctor later reluctantly told the husband and was relieved to find he approved of the doctor's actions and suggested that his wife not be told.

Daniels (1998, p. 78)

It is important to note that two powerful social forces had an impact on the early practice of DI. The morality of the time meant that there was little open discussion of it. The Archbishop of Canterbury established a Commission in 1945 to investigate DI and its report in 1948 (Commission Appointed by His Grace the Archbishop of Canterbury, 1948) opposed DI saying among other things that artificial insemination involved a breach of the marriage and violated the exclusive union set up between husband and wife. To use DI was tantamount to committing adultery. The second powerful force was the stigma associated with infertility and particularly male infertility (Whiteford and Gonzalez, 1995; Nachtigall et al., 1997; Shah, 1999).

As a result of these strong social forces, the practice of DI was known to only a small group of people and most if not all of them did not see it, or want to promote it, as a public issue. Arising out of their concerns about the morality of DI, several church bodies (Catholic Truth Society, 1960; British Council of Churches, 1962) addressed the topic in the 1950s and early 1960s. The topic was, albeit marginally, on the public agenda, but not to the extent that it was viewed as requiring a policy response.

A significant change in the culture of secrecy surrounding AHR occurred as a result of the birth of Louise Brown in 1978. Doctors and scientists associated with IVF were very keen to let the world know of their success and this remains the case. The marvels of medical science's ability to overcome infertility was a very newsworthy topic. With this development came calls for the intervention of governments and for these interventions to cover all areas of AHR, including DI. In New Zealand, for example, a group comprising the Royal Society of New Zealand, the New Zealand Law Society, the Medical Council of New Zealand, the Medical Research Council of New Zealand and the Medical Association of New Zealand requested the Government to appoint a Standing Committee to consider the legal, moral and social issues arising from IVF, artificial insemination by donor and related problems in biotechnology (Royal Society of New Zealand, 1985). Many Western governments did indeed respond to the excitement and anxiety raised by IVF, by establishing committees or commissions to enquire into the scientific and medical advances of human reproduction. Their task was to make recommendations on how governments might intervene in what was seen as a controversial moral area. Such committee recommendations, which Blank (1990, 1998), Walters (1988) and Knoppers and LeBris (1991) have summarized, were primarily concerned with how governments might manage this area, i.e. develop policy. Typical of this need were the terms of reference of the Warnock Committee established in the UK, which included 'to consider what policies and safeguards should be applied which lead to the most comprehensive and what many see as best way of managing the area' (Warnock, 1984).

The Warnock Committee said, after its deliberations, 'perhaps the most important point of agreement the field of inquiry had to cover was that some laws or others needed to be enacted and soon' (Warnock, 1984). In Canada, the Royal Commission on New Reproductive Technologies, set up in 1989 (Royal Commission, 1993), concluded that there was a need for well-defined boundaries in this area and that, within these, account-able regulation was needed to protect the interests of those involved, as well as those of society as a whole. Baird, Chair of the Commission, wrote in 1996, 'Individual decisions regarding the use of reproductive tech-nologies can be personally beneficial yet have undesirable social consequences' (Baird, 1996, p. 107). It is the concern about social conse-quences that leads to public policy.

Haimes has suggested that:

> We need to make connections between the institutions and values of the wider society and the personal needs and concerns of the individuals direct-ly concerned with the practice of donated gametes. We should not lose sight of those individuals and their concerns, but we must also not focus solely on them to the neglect of these wider issues that help to shape their indi-vidual experiences and which they in turn help to shape.
>
> Haimes (1998, p. 68)

The move to a public policy perspective has been problematic and not without its critics. Blank said that 'until the mid-twentieth century, the prac-tice of medicine was largely treated as a private matter between the health professional and the patient' (Blank, 1998b, p. 133). In the area of third-party reproduction and AHR, medical decision-making has been to the fore and the private ordering model has predominated. It is natural to expect that any change to this well-established culture will lead to opposition.

In Sweden there was considerable opposition (Ewerlöf, 1985; Bodgan, 1986; Edvinsson et al., 1990; Hagenfeldt, 1990; Bydgeman, 1991) to the Government move to introduce the Insemination Act in 1984, which required semen providers' identities to be recorded and made available to offspring in the future – should they want this (Sweden, 1984). Daniels and Lalos have suggested, on the basis of their study of the changes that took place, that certain doctors in Sweden sought to sabotage the legisla-tion, as they were so opposed to it (Daniels, 1994; Daniels and Lalos, 1995). Robert Jansen (1999) has expressed considerable concern about Government moves in Canada and the UK to focus increasingly on the public dimensions of AHR. He says, 'society's agents, including physicians, are to be compelled to disregard the personal needs and suffering of cou-ples' and 'why pick out responsible, competent professionals for sanction for responding to what patients want?' and 'we should be explicit about what is happening in Britain, in Canada, and in other countries where ethical decisions affecting individual's reproductive behaviors are being taken by a small group of people and given the imprimatur of government on the grounds of hypothetical harm to society' (Jansen, 1999, p. 13).

It is not only doctors who have expressed concern about what they see as the intrusion of public policy into the private world of medical practice. Charlesworth, a philosopher, argues that in a liberal democratic society, with its strong emphasis on autonomy, 'the right to procreative liberty' should be paramount and legislative prohibitions should not exist' (Charlesworth, 1993). This position has also been adopted by American lawyer John Robertson (1994), who argues for 'procreative freedom'. Both authors, however, acknowledge the limitations of autonomy and procreative freedom. Charlesworth (1993) acknowledges the right of the state to regulate alternative forms of family formation, as it does with adoption, and Robertson (1994) argues for the 'primacy of reproductive freedom in *most* cases'. What seems to be being acknowledged is that public policy should not limit or detract from private decision-making (autonomy), except in certain exceptional cases. Blank and Merrick (1995), on the other hand, claim that: 'State protection of the vulnerable is a key public policy issue.' They have said, 'a major policy objective should be the creation of public mechanisms to protect the interests of all parties, especially those most vulnerable to exploitation and abuse' (Blank and Merrick, 1995, p. 215).

It has to be acknowledged that there is a significant conflict between a commitment to reproductive liberty and a commitment to a consideration of the duties and responsibilities owed to offspring and their families. Drawing on the principle of autonomy, Robertson says, 'As a matter of public policy, the question of secrecy or disclosure to the child is best left to the couple to resolve' (Robertson, 1994, p. 123). This position, however, fails to address the issue of the professional's power and influence over an infertile couple seeking the opportunity to conceive. In all four situations with which this chapter began, the parents were told or advised to keep the nature of the conception a secret. Those who argue for an 'autonomy-based' private ordering model are concerned with the power of the state. It may be that such critics should also question the power of professionals.

Bonnicksen, writing within the American context, has argued for the development of a private policy model to act as a bridge between voluntary ethical principles and mandatory public sector rules. She argues that the private sector should develop rules that are then adhered to by practitioners. She adopts this position because she believes that public action in many areas of biomedicine is unlikely, premature and unwise (Bonnicksen, 1992). Such a position fails to acknowledge the need for laws in certain areas, e.g. the establishment of records in third-party reproduction and to whom and under what circumstances access to those records may be given. Seibel (1996), drawing on the work of Ami Jaeger, lists the US states that have statutes covering DI. This shows that, in 1995, 35 states had statutes relating to DI and 16 did not. Of those with statutes, 20 included a record-keeping requirement and 15 did not. All 35 states with statutes, except one, legitimized the offspring conceived by DI. What is clear from these figures is that, within a federal system of government such as the USA, there can be considerable variation in the legal provisions for DI and third-party reproduction. Blank (1998a) suggests that there are many regulatory options available for, and in use in, DI. These can be placed on a continuum ranging from individual practice to legislation. His continuum includes seven options (Blank, 1998b, p. 134):

- individual clinician
- programme guidelines
- professional association guidelines
- commissions, committees and task forces
- government guidelines
- licensing regulations
- legislation.

Blank suggests that, 'given the complexity of fertility services, it is likely that any activity will involve some combination of these mechanisms' (Blank, 1998b, p. 133). What is clear is that there has been a shift from the previous private ordering or, in Blank's terms, the 'individual clinician' model of decision-taking, to a variety of regulatory options. Different countries have adopted different options. The debate is likely to continue for some time over the available options.

Interest in and concern for the policy dimensions of third-party reproduction have been both recent and, from the point of view of some of the significant stakeholders, controversial. Reaching agreement on an agenda has not been straightforward and this has made policy formation a challenging exercise.

Information sharing in third-party reproduction

Most Western governments have accepted that assisted reproduction should be a concern of public policy makers, and as result set up committees or commissions to investigate and advise them on appropriate action to take. In their review of these reports, Knoppers and LeBris (1991) were able to identify 12 areas of general consensus in these reports. They were also able to identify six areas of disagreement related to cultural, social, economic and religious differences. These differences were: (1) remuneration of donors, (2) access to information by the child, (3) keeping of registers, (4) donation, conservation and experimentation with human embryos, (5) limits on the number of children per donor and (6) genetic diagnosis of embryos. Three of these areas are closely related to the issue of information sharing.

These issues can be seen to revolve around the nature of the relationships between the various involved parties – the parents, the gamete provider, the offspring and the professionals – and in particular what 'information' is shared between these parties. Many of the debates that have occurred relating to the nature of the relationships have used binary/oppositional language such as secrecy and openness (Daniels and Taylor, 1993) and privacy and disclosure (Klock, 1996).

The use of such oppositional language has its limitations, because the options are presented in an either/or format. The use of the term 'information sharing', it is argued, is more helpful in that it recognizes that there may be many degrees of information sharing, and that the sharing may be different with different individuals and at different times (Daniels et al., 1996). It is also less restricting than secrecy and openness, which was often presented as relating to the parents and their offspring only. The last and perhaps most important reason is that the terms 'secrecy' and 'openness' have a strong value connotation which has not always assisted in clarifying the debates and issues surrounding this topic.

The arguments surrounding information sharing have been well rehearsed (Daniels and Taylor, 1993; Leiblum and Aviv, 1997; Blyth and Hunt, 1998) over the past 15–20 years. It is too simplistic to suggest that the opposing views on this issue were, in the early stages, taken by doctors *against* information sharing and counsellors *for* information sharing. Although many may have perceived this as a conflict between disciplines, it is in my view more appropriate to see the conflict as one emerging from differing views of the focus of intervention (treatment). Emerging from the medical model, doctors were more likely to see the infertile couple – and it was almost entirely couples, until relatively recently – as the patients who needed to be 'treated' for the condition of infertility. Those who took a biopsychosocial perspective (Schwartz, 1982; Cook, 1987; Daniels, 2000) or a holistic approach were concerned with the consequences of the 'treatment' and especially the implications for children who would be born. This has led to the debates being presented as putting the needs and rights of the parents against the needs and rights of the child to be born.

Recent work formulates the issue as a 'treatment of infertility model' and a 'family building model' (Daniels, 2002). The shift to a family focus is important in that it centres attention on the well-being of both the parents and the offspring. Again it is not helpful to present the two models as oppositional, but rather it is necessary to recognize that the use of third-party reproduction involves both. The specialists in each of the models need to collaborate closely to ensure the well-being of future families. As infertility requires medical assessment and treatment, it is of course the medical perspective and model that become dominant. One of the conflicts, however, is that the 'building a family' perspective is also perceived as being subject to the medical perspective, e.g. doctors advising parents not to tell the child about how she or he was conceived. In fact the vast majority of issues that arise for families who have used third-party reproduction are social, psychological, ethical and perhaps legal (McWhinnie, 1992; Dudley and Neave, 1997; Blyth et al., 1998). In these areas, the doctor is not perceived as the specialist with expert knowledge. Having made this generalization, it remains important to acknowledge that some doctors have developed considerable knowledge and expertise in this area.

It is partly against this backdrop that certain jurisdictions have acted, or are considering acting, to focus on the psychosocial needs of children and their families. In Sweden, the decision to introduce their legislation (Swedish Law on Artificial Insemination 1984) was occasioned by the social father of a child conceived as a result of DI, who sought and won release from his parental responsibilities on the grounds that he was sterile. As the semen provider was unknown, the child became legally 'fatherless'. The case highlighted the need for provision to be made to protect the child's rights and needs. Those who argued for the rights and needs of children were opposed by those (mainly doctors) who wanted to maintain the established system. Doctors in Sweden (Bogdan, 1986; Bydgeman, 1989), for example, argue that, if it were possible for children conceived by DI to have access to identification of 'their' gamete provider, it would mean the end of the service – in other words treating infertility was the dominant focus and all else was placed in a secondary position. It seems that those who argue for the 'family building' perspective, and the rights and needs of Geraldine, Rebecca, Bill and Susannah and their families, have increasingly had to advocate that governments must intervene in this area to protect their vulnerable citizens and families.

The legislation that has been enacted in this area has usually involved the establishment of registers in which the names of the involved parties are recorded. Provisions have been made as to by whom, when and how access can be gained to these registers. In the four jurisdictions cited earlier, Austria, Sweden, Switzerland and the State of Victoria in Australia, access can be obtained by offspring, whereas in the UK access to information on the registers is very limited and subject to stringent controls (Human Fertilisation and Embryology Act 1990). The registers, of course, record information only from the time of their establishment. This leaves those born before the advent of registers unable to access information. In response to this issue, the State of Victoria in Australia has become the first government to establish a Voluntary Register. The Register provides for those who are seeking or offering information to be possibly linked.

Other 'registers' exist, in the form of hospital clinic or practitioner records. In a number of cases known to the author (in several different countries), individuals conceived as a result of DI have been able to access such records. This has been possible because some clinics have made contact with previous semen providers to ask them whether they would be prepared to provide information and/or possibly have contact. In several instances, this has been achieved only as a result of persistent applications by DI offspring, aided by advocacy from concerned staff.

The establishment and maintenance of a register are matters for governments, as already happens with births, deaths and marriages, and adoptions. Without registers, either government or clinic based, there is no possibility of obtaining what might eventuate to be vital medical information, not to mention the psychosocial needs identified by the individuals at the beginning of the chapter. It also needs to be acknowledged that, as a result of the 'genetic revolution', information concerning parentage will become increasingly accessible with, as yet, little thought being given to the consequences.

It is of note that New Zealand, which has not as yet enacted any legislation concerning registers and provision for information sharing, has perhaps the most progressive approach to information sharing. One of the main indications of this is that semen or egg providers will not be recruited unless they are prepared to be identified to offspring in the future. Counsellors see virtually all individuals or couples seeking third-party reproduction and issues associated with information sharing are very fully explored. A study by Adair (1999) of the experiences of 181 New Zealand parents, who had created their families through DI, showed significantly that 30 per cent of the parents had already told their children about their DI origins. It was more important that, of the parents who had not yet told their children, a further 77 per cent reported that they did intend to impart this information to their offspring in the future (Adair, 1999). Registers are currently kept in clinics, but legislation is soon to be introduced that will see this formalized in law.

In contrasting the experiences in Sweden and New Zealand, I would suggest that the Swedish policy was based on the expectation that legislation would lead to a change in the way professionals and parents behaved. A recent study of parents who had given birth to a child with the assistance of DI, after the Swedish legislation in 1985, showed that most parents (89 per cent) had not informed their child (Gottlieb et al., 2000).

However, 52 per cent of parents had either told the children (11 per cent) or stated in their response that they were intending to tell them – many of the children were still quite young. A total of 59 per cent of couples stated that they had told someone else and in most cases this was a close family member. Through this research, Gottlieb and colleagues highlight that compliance with the intentions of the legislation are regarded as low, even though the number of parents willing to inform their child is high when viewed from an international perspective.

The New Zealand experience, which has been influenced by many factors, was based on an educational approach (Daniels, 1999). Legislation has therefore followed changes in practice, rather than, as happened in Sweden, being intended to produce change. It is not appropriate to think that it is an either/or situation; rather it should be emphasized that changes of law that are not accompanied by changes of attitude will have only minimal impact on changed practice.

It is of note that two countries – the UK and Canada – are currently considering these issues. Canada's proposed legislation (Canada, Proposals for Legislation 2001) states in its preamble: 'The Parliament of Canada appreciates the paramount need for measures to protect the best interests of children affected by the application of these technologies.' Having made this commitment, the Bill then restricts access to information by offspring conceived via third-party reproduction. In effect the proposed legislation will protect the gamete provider's anonymity, thus giving their interests a higher priority than those of the offspring. Such a position represents a continuation of the traditional approach to information sharing in third-party reproduction, and seems to be based on the advocacy of one of the stakeholders – the medical profession. The voices of other stakeholders, most notably some offspring and their parents who have taken a public stance, have been heard, but have often been dismissed as unrepresentative. This may reflect the stage of consciousness-raising in Canada on this topic. One of the difficulties with any legislation – whatever it covers – is that it is unlikely to be reviewed or changed for some time. In the UK, the Department of Health released a discussion paper on 21 December 2001, inviting submissions on whether the current policy of donor anonymity and no access by offspring should be continued or changed.

The advent of the consumer group movement in third-party reproduction has played, and continues to play, a significant role in the consideration of information sharing. This movement, with its strong bases in New Zealand, Australia, Canada, Sweden and the UK, has become increasingly active in advocating for government action in these areas. Representing families (and often including gamete providers in their membership) who have been participants in third-party reproduction, they have an important message to share. They do not of course represent

all such families but, given that they have joined forces – and thus rejected the privacy and secrecy often associated with their family formation –
they have ensured that the issues are very firmly on the public agenda.
Their advocacy for changes in the traditional way in which DI has been
practised has to be listened to – they are after all vital stakeholders. Even
more vital, however, are the offspring – the main stakeholder, it could be
argued – who want to see policies formulated and enacted that recognize
their needs and rights. As Snowden points out, with the passing of time
and the ageing of offspring (becoming adults), such people will become
their own best advocates in pressing for change that allows them to argue
for the right to genetic information about themselves (Snowden, 1998).
In the four years since Snowden wrote, there have been an increasing
number of adult offspring acting as their own advocates. Their contribution to policy development is and will be extremely powerful.

Challenges to the policy of secrecy in third-party reproduction have, in
the main, been driven by concerns for children and, more recently, families. The move towards information sharing, especially in the four
jurisdictions that have enacted legislation embracing this policy, has an
impact on the providers of the gametes and it is to them that we now turn.
The removal of the traditional anonymity of semen providers, in particular, but also oocyte providers, was predicted to be a major disaster; Beck
(1984) said: 'If there is no anonymity then there will be no DI. In addition, we have a definite responsibility to the donor, which would be
jeopardized with disclosure of the process. There will be no more AID
anywhere if the donor thinks his privacy and his protection are threatened' (Beck, 1984, p. 194). The gamete provider is an indispensable part
of third-party reproduction – without his or her contribution there would
be no third-party reproduction. The impact of policies that remove
provider anonymity therefore needs to be considered.

Until recently, little was known about the providers of gametes. It was
thought that the main reason for this was that doctors wished to 'protect'
the semen providers from public scrutiny, as well as maintaining the low
public profile of DI and third-party reproduction. In 1964, Finegold
(1964, p. 35) said, 'It is generally agreed that the donor's identity should
be veiled in absolute obscurity', and Glezerman (1981) said that the
semen from a provider should be seen as 'material from an anonymous
testis' with the donor being actually a 'non-person'. However, from the
early 1980s, semen providers began as a result of studies to be able to
'speak for themselves', resulting in the emergence of a different picture
(Daniels, 1998). A study in Australia (Nicholas and Tyler, 1983) reported
that 56 per cent of men in their study supported the idea of a national register of names and addresses of providers and recipients. Rowland (1983)
also found that 60 per cent of the semen providers whom she interviewed

said that they would not mind meeting with the 'child' at the age of 18. For a review of the studies of semen providers from 1980 to 1997, see Daniels (1998). The evidence from these studies indicates that the situation from the semen provider's point of view is not as black and white as had been previously portrayed, and that a proportion of semen providers did not see anonymity as a prerequisite for contributing semen.

Of major importance in the debates about donor anonymity is the investigation of what has happened to gamete provider recruitment and availability after the introduction of requirements about the registration of names and provider details. The only study that is available in this respect is the one conducted by Daniels and Lalos (1995), which showed that after the introduction of the Swedish legislation in 1985 there was an initial decline in the number of available semen providers. At the time of the study in 1994, however, more semen providers were available than before the legislation. Some differences in the characteristics of men becoming semen providers after the legislation were in evidence. The most notable of these was the age of the men – they were older. In New Zealand, where for the past 10 years the policy and practice of clinics have been only to recruit gamete providers who were prepared to be identified to offspring in the future (should they wish this), the number of providers has remained stable. No specific studies measuring the actual numbers in New Zealand have been undertaken, it should be noted.

It is also important to note that the impact of national policies, whether codified in legislation or developed as a result of professional practice, may be only one factor determining gamete provider attitudes. In a study by Daniels and colleagues (1996) of semen providers in two London clinics, it was found that the comparisons between the policies of the two clinics showed that motivations were related to social positioning and location at the time of donation, e.g. payment was a motivating factor for younger men who were students and viewed providing semen as a source of income, in comparison to the other group who were older, married with children of their own, and had heard about DI through a medical person or the media and decided to contribute because of a desire to help others. The policies that a clinic therefore develops in relation to recruitment are likely to impact on the types and attitudes of those who respond.

In countries such as Australia and New Zealand many clinics will seek to trace semen providers – if records still exist – if they receive enquiries from offspring. Such contact with the providers is in the first instance to ascertain whether they are prepared to share information or perhaps contact. This protects the undertakings given to providers at the time that they supplied semen. Again, no evidence is available on the use of, or results from, such endeavours. The main reason for this is the relatively recent advent of clinics prepared to adopt a mediating role. A British semen gamete provider with whom I have had several discussions has pointed out that when he was 'recruited' he was told that anonymity was required and that his privacy would be protected. He happily accepted this as appropriate. Now, as a married man with two children (11 and 9), he sees the contribution of semen in a different way and recognizes the importance of information about him being available to any offspring – should they want this. With this in mind he wrote to the Harley Street Clinic in London (where he provided his semen), offering to be available should they receive any requests from offspring. His offer was declined, the clinic stating that they did not do that sort of thing. He later wrote to the HFEA in the UK where his offer was rejected, as the HFEA had no system for managing such offers.

The move to information sharing is likely to continue to have an impact on gamete providers. As the authors pointed out, 'a man is a sperm donor for only a short time; after that he is a man with children in someone else's family' (Purdie et al., 1994). Those children, when mature, may well want information about 'their' semen provider. A great deal of policy, and in fact legislation, in France (Bioethics Act, 1994) is based on the premiss that the man or woman is a provider of gametes only and that they need have no concerns or responsibilities regarding the well-being of the offspring and the families they have helped to create. Evidence from the studies in DI referred to above and in oocyte donation (Sauer et al., 1994; Soderstrom-Anttila, 1995) indicate that many gamete providers do not see their 'gift of life' in this way. Certainly, offspring who know of the nature of their conception – such as those mentioned at the outset of this chapter – do not want 'their' providers to take this view. Parents of offspring likewise are also challenging the anonymity of gamete providers (Brewaeys et al., 1997; Blyth, 1999; Baetens et al., 2000) and calling for policies that embrace the well-being and best interests of all the parties involved in third-party reproduction.

Conclusion

In the past, the best interests of some parties have been pitched against the best interests of other parties. In the main it has been professionals, in many cases through their influence on policy makers, who have determined that it should be so. Evidence presented in this chapter shows that an alternative model, which serves the interests of all, is possible, but that the adoption of such an approach falls most appropriately in the realm of public policy. What is clear is that there are those who would not, in the interests of reproductive liberty and freedom, want to have public policy in this area. Such a position, primarily because it does not afford protection to those who are vulnerable and for whom states see themselves as having a responsibility, is becoming increasingly unacceptable. Different countries are at varying points in relation to their particular policy development. The problem has, however, been identified. The calls for agenda setting, policy formation, adoption and implementation continue to be conflictual, and managing such conflict remains a major challenge.

References

Adair V (1999) Telling the story: parents' scripts for donor offspring. Human Reproduction 14: 1392–1399.

Anderson JE (1990) Public Policy-Making: An introduction. Boston: Houghton Mifflin.

Baetens P, Devroey P, Camus M, Van Steirteghem AC, Ponjaert-Kristofferson I (2000) Counselling couples and donors for oocyte donation: the decision to use either known or anonymous oocytes. Human Reproduction 15: 476–484.

Baird P (1996) Ethical issues of fertility and reproduction. Annual Review of Medicine 47: 107–16.

Beck WW (1984) Two hundred years of artificial insemination. Fertility and Sterility 14: 194.

Blank RH (1990) Regulating Reproduction. New York: Columbia University Press.

Blank RH (1998) Regulation of donor insemination. In: Daniels KR, Haimes E (eds), Donor Insemination: International social science perspectives. Cambridge: Cambridge University Press.

Blank R, Merrick JC (1995) Human Reproduction: Emerging technologies and conflicting rights. Washington DC: CQ Press.

Blizzard J (1977) Blizzard and the Holy Ghost. London: Peter Owen.

Blyth E (1999) Secrets and lies: barriers to the exchange of genetic origins information following donor assisted conception. Adoption and Fostering 23: 49–58.

Blyth E, Hunt J (1998) Sharing genetic origins information in donor assisted conception: views from licensed centres on HFEA donor information. Human Reproduction 13: 3274–3277.

Blyth E, Crawshaw M, Speirs J (eds) (1998) Truth and the Child Ten Years On: Information exchange in donor assisted conception. Birmingham: British Association of Social Workers.

Bogdan M (1986) Artificial Insemination in Swedish Law. Comparative Law Year Book 10: 91–106.

Bonnicksen AL (1992) Human embryos and genetic testing: a private policy model. Politics and the Life Sciences 11: 53–63.

Brewaeys A (2001) Review: parent–child relationships and child development in donor insemination families. Human Reproduction 7: 38–46.

Brewaeys A, Golombok S, Naaktgeboren N, de Bruyn J, Van Hall E (1997) Donor insemination: Dutch parents' opinions about confidentiality and donor anonymity and the emotional adjustment of their child. Human Reproduction 12: 1591–1597.

British Council of Churches (1962) Human Reproduction: A study of some emergent problems in the light of the Christian Faith. London: British Council of Churches.

Bydgeman M (1989) Swedish law concerning insemination. IPPF Medical Bulletin 23: 3–4.

Bydgeman M (1991) The Swedish Insemination Act. Acta Obstetrica et Gynecologica Scandinavica 70: 265–266.

Canada (2001) Proposals for Legislation Governing Assisted Human Reproduction. Health Canada.

Catholic Truth Society (1960) Artificial Insemination: Evidence on behalf of the Catholic Body in England and Wales. London: Catholic Truth Society.

Charlesworth M (1993) Bioethics in a Liberal Society. Cambridge: Cambridge University Press.

Commission Appointed by His Grace the Archbishop of Canterbury (1948) Artificial Human Insemination. London: Society for the Propagation of Christian Knowledge.

Cook EP (1987) Characteristics of the biopsychosocial crisis of infertility. Journal of Counselling and Development 65: 465–70.

Daniels KR (1994) The Swedish Insemination Act and its impact. Australian New Zealand Journal of Obstetrics and Gynecology 34: 437–439.

Daniels KR (1998) The semen providers. In: Daniels KR, Haimes E (eds), Donor Insemination: International social science perspectives. Cambridge: Cambridge University Press.

Daniels KR (1999) Donor Insemination in New Zealand: from early beginnings to the millennium. Pathways. New Zealand Infertility Society, pp. 6–9.

Daniels KR (2000) Infertility treatment: a biopsychosocial perspective. Orgyn 2000: 11–14.

Daniels KR (2002) Towards a family approach for donor insemination. Journal of Obstetrics and Gynaecology of Canada 24: 17–21.

Daniels KR, Haimes E (eds) (1998) Donor Insemination: International social science perspectives. Cambridge: Cambridge University Press.

Daniels KR, Lalos O (1995) The Swedish Insemination Act and the availability of donors. Human Reproduction 10: 1871–1874.

Daniels KR, Taylor K (1993) Secrecy and openness in donor insemination. Politics and the Life Sciences 12: 155–170.

Daniels KR, Curson R, Lewis GM (1996) Families formed as a result of semen donor insemination: the views of semen donors. Child and Family Social Work 1: 97–106.

Dudley M, Neave G (1997) Issues for families and children where conception was achieved using donor gametes, let the offspring speak: Discussions on donor conception. Sydney, New South Wales, The Donor Conception Support Group of Australia, Inc., pp. 125– 36.

Edvinsson A, Forsman L, Milson I, Nordfors G (1990) Givarinsemination vid Manlig Infertilitet: Slut pa en Epok? [Donor Insemination for male infertility: the end of an era?] Lakartidningen 87: 1871–1872.

Ewerlöf G (1985) Artificial insemination – legislation and debate. Current Sweden (329).

Finegold WJ (1964) Artificial Insemination. Springfield, Ill: Charles C Thomas.

Glezerman M (1981) Two hundred and seventy cases of artificial donor insemination: management and results. Fertility and Sterility 35: 180–187.

Gottlieb C, Lalos O, Lindblad F (2000) Disclosure of donor insemination to the child: the impact of Swedish legislation on couples' attitudes. Human Reproduction 15: 2052–2056.

Hagenfeldt K (1990) Givarinsemination: Behandlingsmetod i Kris. [Donor insemination: a treatment in crisis.] Lakartidningen 87: 1849–1850.

Haimes E (1998) The making of 'the DI child': changing representations of people conceived through donor insemination. In: Daniels KR, Haimes E (eds), Donor Insemination: International social science perspectives. Cambridge: Cambridge University Press.

Hamilton, G (2001) Documentary New Zealand, Are You my Father? TVNZ, Monday 10 September 8.30pm.

Hewitt G (2001) Family Matters – Birth Rights. Compass. ABC TV 5 August 2001.

Human Fertilisation and Embryology Authority (2000) The Patient's Guide to DI. London: HFEA.

Jansen R (1999) Brave new ethics. Orgyn 11–15.

Klock SC (1996) Privacy and disclosure in infertility treatment. Psychotherapy in Practice 2: 55–71.

Knoppers BM, LeBris S (1991) Recent advances in medically assisted conception: legal ethical and social issues. American Journal of Law and Medicine 18: 329–361.

Leiblum SR, Aviv AL (1997) Disclosure issues and decisions of couples who conceived via donor insemination. Journal of Psychosomatic Obstetrics and Gynaecology 18: 292–300.

McWhinnie AM (1992) Creating children – the medical and social dilemmas of assisted reproduction. Adoption and Fostering 16: 29–39.

Mills CW (1970) The Sociological Imagination. Harmondsworth: Penguin.

Nachtigall RD, Tschann JM, Szkupinski Quiroga S, Pitcher L, Becker G (1997) Stigma, disclosure, and family functioning among parents of children conceived through donor insemination. Fertility and Sterility 68: 83–89.

Nicholas MK, Tyler PP (1983) Characteristics, attitudes and personalities of AI donors. Clinical Reproduction and Fertility 2: 389–396.

Purdie A, Peek C, Adair V, Graham F, Fisher R (1994) Attitudes of parents of young children to sperm donation – implications for donor recruitment. Human Reproduction 9: 1355–1358.

Robertson JA (1994) Children of Choice: Freedom and the new reproductive technologies. Princeton: Princeton University Press.

Rowland R (1983) Attitudes and opinions of donors on an artificial insemination by donor (AID) programme. Clinical Reproduction and Fertility 2: 249–259.

Rowland R (1984) Social and psychological consequences of secrecy in artificial insemination by donor. In: Adoption and AID: Access to information? Melbourne: Monash University Centre for Human Bioethics.

Royal Commission on New Reproductive Technologies (1993) Proceed With Care: Final Report of the Royal Commission on New Reproductive Technologies. Canada: Minister of Government Services.

Royal Society of New Zealand (1985) Issues arising from in vitro fertilisation, artificial insemination by donor and related problems in biotechnology. New Zealand Medical Journal 98: 396–398.

Sauer M, Ary BR, Paulson R (1994) The demographic characterisation of women participating in oocyte donation: a review of 300 consecutively performed cycles. International Journal of Obstetrics and Gynaecology 45: 147–151.

Schwartz GE (1982) Testing the biopsychosocial model: the ultimate challenge facing behavioral medicine? Journal of Consulting and Clinical Psychology 50: 1040–1053.

Seibel MM (1996) Therapeutic donor insemination. In: Seibel MM, Crockin SL (eds), Family Building Through Egg and Sperm Donation. Sudbury: Jones & Bartlett Publishers.

Shah R (1999) Psychological impact of infertility on men. In: Jansen R, Mortimer D (eds), Towards Reproductive Certainty: Fertility and genetics beyond 1999. New York: Parthenon, pp. 28–36.

Snowden R (1998) Psychosocial discontinuities introduced by the new reproductive technologies. Journal of Community and Applied Social Psychology 8: 249–259.

Soderstrom-Anttila V (1995) Follow-up study of Finnish volunteer oocyte donors, concerning their attitudes to oocyte donation. Human Reproduction 10: 3073–3076.

Walters LR (1988) Ethical aspects of the new reproductive technologies. Annals of the New York Academy of Sciences 646–663.

Walters N (2000) Too much knowledge is a dad thing. The Independent 7: 7.

Warnock M (1984) Report of the Committee of Inquiry into Human Fertilization and Embryology. London: HMSO.

Warnock M (1985) Moral thinking and government policy: The Warnock Committee on Human Embryology. Milbank Memorial Fund Quarterly Health and Society 63: 504–522.

Whiteford LM, Gonzalez L (1995) Stigma: the hidden burden of infertility. Social Science and Medicine 40: 27–36.

Resources

British Agency for Adoption and Fostering (BAAF)
Skyline House
200 Union Street
London SE1 OLY
Tel: 020 7593 2000 (HQ)
Fax: 020 7593 2001
Helpline: 020 7593 2060
Website: www.baaf.org.uk
Gives information and advice, produces information leaflets and books including *Adoption and Fostering Journal.*

British Fertility Society (BFS)
British Fertility Society Secretariat
16 The Courtyard
Woodlands
Bradley Stoke
Bristol BS32 4NQ
Tel: 01454 642217
Fax: 01454 642222
Website: www.britishfertilitysociety.com
E-mail: bsf@bioscientifica.com
Professional newsletter and journal: *Human Fertility*

British Infertility Counsellors Association (BICA)
69 Division Street
Sheffield S1 4GE
Tel: 01342 843880
Website: www.bica.net
Professional journal: *Journal of Fertility Counselling*

The British Psychological Society (BPS)
St Andrews House
48 Princess Road East
Leicester LE1 7DR
Tel: 0116 254 9568
Fax: 0116 247 0787
E-mail: mail@bps.org.uk
Website: www.bps.org.uk
Professional journal: *The Psychologist*
Lists chartered, clinical and counselling psychologists.

CHILD – The National Infertility Support Network
Charter House
43 St Leonards Road
Bexhill-on-Sea
East Sussex TN40 1JA
Tel: 01424 732361
Fax:01424 731858
E-mail: office@email2.child.org.uk
Website: www.child.org.uk
National self-help network offering information and support for those trying for a family, carry books on the subject.

COTS (Childlessness Overcome Through Surrogacy)
Loandhu Cottage
Gruids
Lairg
Sutherland
Scotland IV27 4EF
Tel: 01549 402401
Information line: 0906 680 0088
E-mail: cotsuk@enterprise.net
www.surrogacy.org.uk
Agency specializing in surrogacy arrangements, provides information and counselling.

Donor Conception (DC) Network
PO Box 265
Sheffield S3 7YX
Tel/Fax: 020 8245 4369
E-mail: dcnetwork@appleonline.net
Website: www.dcnetwork.org
Group of parents using DI treatment and/or whose children were born from donated gametes, sperm or eggs. Offers practical and emotional support to parents about telling their children about their origins, and enables parents and children to meet others in a similar position. Offshoot: Single Women Insemination Group (SWIG).

FORESIGHT (Association for the Promotion of Pre-Conceptual Care)
28 The Paddock
Godalming
Surrey GU7 1XD
Tel: 01483 427839
Fax: 01483 427668
Offers a video, booklets and leaflets on non-technological approaches to fertility issues

Human Fertilisation and Embryology Authority (HFEA)
Paxton House
30 Artillery Lane
London E1 7LS
Tel: 020 7377 5077
Fax: 020 7377 1871
Website: www.hfea.gov.uk
Statutory body responsible for licensing fertility clinics in the UK. Produces information leaflets and list of clinics.

ISSUE (The National Fertility Association)
114 Lichfield Street
Walsall WS1 1SZ
Tel: 01922 722888
Website: www.issue.co.uk
National fertility support organization, provides advice, information and support about infertility treatments and services; regional support groups and regular newsletter.

Miscarriage Association
c/o Clayton Hospital
Northgate, Wakefield
West Yorkshire WF1 3JS
Tel: 01924 200799
Fax: 01924 298834
Website: www.the-ma.org.uk

National Egg and Embryo Donation Society (NEEDS)
Department of Reproductive Medicine
Regional IVF Unit
St Mary's Hospital
Whitworth Park
Manchester M13 0JH
Tel: 0161 276 6000
Fax: 0161 224 0957

National Gamete Donation Trust
PO Box 137
Manchester M13 0YX
Tel: 0161 276 6000
Website: www.ngdt.org.uk

National Infertility Awareness Campaign (NIAC)
PO Box 2106
London W1A 3D2
Tel: 020 7439 3067
Website: www.repromed.co.uk/NIAC/info/

Nuffield Council of Bioethics
28 Bedford Square
London WC1B 3JS
Tel: 020 7681 1619
Fax: 020 7637 1712
Website: www.nuffieldbioethics.org

Post Adoption Centre
8 Torriano Mews
Torriano Avenue
London NW5 2RZ
Tel: 020 7284 0555
Fax: 020 7482 2367
Website: www.postadoptioncentre.org.uk
Training organization and confidential counselling service for anyone involved in adoption.

Twins and Multiple Birth Foundation (TAMBA)
Queen Charlotte's and Chelsea Hospital
Du Cane Road
London W12 0HS
Tel: 020 8383 3519
Fax: 020 8383 3041
E-mail mbf@ic.ac.uk
Website: www.multiplebirths.org.uk

Europe

European Society for Human Reproduction and Embryology (ESHRE)
Central Office
Van Akenstraat 41
B-1850 Grimbergen
Belgium
Tel: +32 02 269 09 69
Fax: +32 02 269 56 00
E-mail: eshre@pophost.eunet.be
Website: www.eshre.com

North America

American Fertility Society (AFS)
1209 Montgomery Highway
Birmingham AL. 35216-2809, USA
Tel: +1 315 724 4348
International association of professionals with special interest in fertility.

American Holistic Medical Association
4101 Lake Boone Trail
Raleigh NC 27607, USA
Tel: + 1 919 787 5181

American Society for Reproductive Medicine (ASRM)
Suite 203
408 12th Street SW
Washington DC 20024-2125, USA
Tel: +1 212 863 2439
Fax: +1 212 484 4039
Website: www.asrm.com
Organization for professionals in reproductive health, providing pamphlets on range of topics. Professional Journal: *Fertility and Sterility*.

Association for Prenatal and Perinatal Psychology and Health
340 Colony Road
Box 994
Geyserville
California CA 95441-0994, USA
Tel: +1 707 857 4041

International Council on Infertility Information Dissemination (Inciid)
PO Box 6836
Arlington VA 22206, USA
Tel: +1 703 379 9178
Fax: +1 703 379 1593
Website: www.inciid.org

Infertility Network
160 Pickering Street
Toronto
Ontario M4E 3JT
Canada
Website: www.InfertilityNetwork.org

Organization of Parents Through Surrogacy (OPTS) National Headquarters
PO Box 611
Gurnee IL 60031, USA
Tel: +1 847 782 0224
Fax: +1 847 782 0240
Website: www.opts.com
National non-profit organization run by volunteers providing mutual support, networking and information including directory of agencies, attorneys, physicians and psychological professionals plus newsletter.

RESOLVE Inc.
1310 Broadway
Somerville MA 02144-1731
Business office +1 617 623 1156
Fax: +1 617 623 0252
Helpline: +1 617 623 0744
Website: www.resolve.org
Provides education, support and advocacy services with chapters nationwide.

Australia

ACCESS (Australia National Infertility Network)
PO Box 959
Parramatta
New South Wales 2124, Australia
Tel: +61 2 9670 2380
Consumer association providing advice, advocacy and fact sheets.

Australian Multiple Birth Foundation (AMBA)
PO Box 914
Glen Waverley 3150, Australia

Donor Conception Support Group
PO Box 53
George's Hall
New South Wales 2198, Australia
Tel: +61 2 9435 0976

Infertility Treatment Authority (ITA)
30/570 Bourke Street
Melbourne 3000
Tel: +61 4 8601 5250

Melbourne IVF
10/320 Victoria Parade
East Melbourne
Victoria 3002, Australia
Tel: +61 3 9473 4444
Fax: +61 3 9473 4454

Websites

AceBabes
www.acebabes.co.uk
A network for families after successful assisted human reproduction.

Adoption International
www.rainbowkids.com

American Infertility Association
www.americaninfertility.org
Fact sheet – talking with children about ovum donation.

American Surrogacy Centre
www.surrogacy.com
Online group offering information and support, including information on egg donation.

Assisted Conception and Infertility Research Network
www.hud.ac.uk/hhs/research/acirg/network.htm
Contact point for researchers from a range of backgrounds.

Assisted Human Reproduction Bibliographic Database
http://ahr.sowk.canterbury.ac.nz
Nearly 4000 entries searchable by title, author, keywords and abstracts compiled by Ken Daniels.

BioNews
www.progress.org.uk
Progress Educational Trust
140 Gray's Inn Road
London WC1X 8AX
Free weekly news digest of top stories in AHR and human genetics.

The Bertarelli Foundation
www.bertarelli.edu
Foundation created to promote and improve understanding of the many aspects of infertility.

Child of My Dreams
www.child-dream.com
Includes articles, message boards and chat groups.

Daisy Network: Premature Menopause Support Group
www.daisynetwork.org

Donor Offspring
www.donoroffspring.com

Enhancement Technologies Group
www.gene.ucl.ac.uk/bioethics/index.html

The Fertility Network
www.ivf.net

Human Fertility
www.srf-reproduction.org/journal/humanfertility

ManNotIncluded.com Ltd
Prince Consort House
Albert Embankment
London SE1 7TG
138 Harley St
London W1G 7LA
Tel: 0870 420 2566
www.mannotincluded.com

More to Life
www.moretolife.co.uk

ReproMed
www.repromed.net/gateway/Patient_Support_Organisations
Developed by ISSUE to provide reports for involuntarily childless people.

Society for the Study of Fertility
www.ssf.org.uk
Includes access to abstracts of *Journal of Reproduction and Fertility*.

TOLI (Time of Life International) UK
www.toli.org.uk

World Health Organization
www.who.org

Worldwide Fertility Network
www.ferti.net

Index